SOCIAL EXPERIENCES OF BREASTFEEDING

Building bridges between research, policy and practice

Edited by
Sally Dowling, David Pontin
and Kate Boyer

GW00578140

P

First published in Great Britain in 2018 by

Policy Press
University of Bristol
1-9 Old Park Hill
Bristol
BS2 8BB
UK
t: +44 (0)117 954 5940
pp-info@bristol.ac.uk
www.policypress.co.uk

North America office:
Policy Press
c/o The University of Chicago Press
1427 East 60th Street
Chicago, IL 60637, USA
t: +1 773 702 7700
f: +1 773-702-9756
sales@press.uchicago.edu
www.press.uchicago.edu

© Policy Press 2018

British Library Cataloguing in Publication Data
A catalogue record for this book is available from the British Library

Library of Congress Cataloging-in-Publication Data
A catalog record for this book has been requested

ISBN 978-1-4473-3850-5 paperback
ISBN 978-1-4473-3849-9 hardcover
ISBN 978-1-4473-3852-9 ePub
ISBN 978-1-4473-3853-6 Mobi
ISBN 978-1-4473-3851-2 ePdf

The right of Sally Dowling, David Pontin and Kate Boyer to be identified as editors of this work has been asserted by them in accordance with the Copyright, Designs and Patents Act 1988.

Cover design by Qube Design
Front cover image: Unicef UK/Mead
Printed and bound in Great Britain by CMP, Poole
Policy Press uses environmentally responsible print partners

We would like to dedicate this book to the memory of Miriam Labbok (1949–2016). Sally and David met her at the Breastfeeding and Feminism events in Chapel Hill, North Carolina, and were both inspired and encouraged by her. Her energy, wisdom and knowledge will be greatly missed by everyone involved in breastfeeding research, policy and practice.

Contents

List of tables and figures

Tables

Figures

Notes on contributors

Alison Bartlett teaches at the University of Western Australia. She has an enduring interest in understanding breastfeeding as a cultural practice, and has published widely on the topic, including her book *Breastwork: Rethinking breastfeeding* (2005), and an edited volume, *Giving breast milk: Body ethics and contemporary breastfeeding practice* (2010), with Rhonda Shaw. Her most recent work on materiality and social memory is *Things that liberate: An Australian feminist Wunderkammer* (2013), edited with Margaret Henderson.

Maia Boswell-Penc is an author, sustainability educator, workshop and retreat facilitator, and consultant. Previously, as faculty in the Department of Women's, Gender and Sexuality Studies at the State University of New York in Albany, she taught environmental, social justice, diversity, human sexuality and interpersonal development courses. In addition to publishing articles in environmental studies, women's studies, diversity studies, disability studies, and studies in racism and critical theory, she has published *Tainted milk: Breastmilk, feminisms and the politics of environmental degradation* (2006). She is currently working on a book about climate change and compassion.

Kate Boyer is a Senior Lecturer in Feminist Geography in the School of Geography and Planning at Cardiff University. She received her PhD from McGill University, Montreal, in 2001 and has been working in the UK since 2007. She has published on breastfeeding in public, combining lactation with wage work, breastmilk donation and breastfeeding activism, and presented research on women's experiences of breastfeeding in the UK (with Sally Dowling) to the All Party Parliamentary Group on Infant Feeding and Inequalities at the Houses of Parliament, London, in 2016. In 2018 Kate published the book *Spaces and politics of motherhood* (Rowman and Littlefield International).

Amy Brown is a Professor in the Department of Public Health, Policy and Social Sciences at Swansea University, UK, where she leads the MSc in Child Public Health. She has published over 60 papers exploring psychological, cultural and societal barriers to breastfeeding. Her primary focus explores how to shift our perception of breastfeeding as an individual mothering issue to a wider public health problem, considering how we can create a society that protects and encourages breastfeeding. She is author of *Breastfeeding uncovered: Who really decides* *how we feed our babies*, *The positive breastfeeding book* and *Why starting solids matters*, all published by Pinter and Martin ltd.

Louise Condon has an academic background in child welfare and social policy, and is Professor of Nursing at Swansea University. When her own children were small, Louise was a National Childbirth Trust breastfeeding counsellor, an experience which has shaped much of her future career. As a midwife, health visitor and then public health manager, Louise has been concerned with supporting breastfeeding mothers in the community and at a strategic level. Her research interests are in health inequalities and health promotion, and she is an editor of *Health Expectations*.

Sally Dowling is Senior Lecturer in Adult Nursing at the University of the West of England (UWE), Bristol. Her academic background is in the social sciences and public health; she worked for 21 years in National Health Service (NHS) posts in a range of settings. The motivation for her PhD was her own experience of breastfeeding her youngest two daughters well beyond the current norms in the UK. She has published on breastfeeding in public, stigma and breastfeeding, long-term breastfeeding, and breastfeeding and liminality. She is currently working on several projects looking at breast milk sharing, including editing a special issue of *Maternal and Child Nutrition* (with Tanya Cassidy and Fiona Dykes). She is Associate Editor for *International Breastfeeding Journal* and on the editorial board of Sociological Research Online.

Fiona Dykes is Professor of Maternal and Infant Health; she established and leads the Maternal and Infant Nutrition and Nurture Unit (MAINN) at the University of Central Lancashire and convenes the MAINN Conference, held biannually in the UK and on alternate years overseas. The editorial office for the journal *Maternal and Child Nutrition* is situated in MAINN, and Fiona is a member of the editorial board. She is an Adjunct Professor at Western Sydney University and holds Visiting Professorships at Högskolan Dalarna, Sweden, and the Chinese University of Hong Kong. Her interests include the global, sociocultural and political influences upon infant and young child feeding practices, with expertise in ethnography and other qualitative research methods. Fiona is author of 80+ peer-reviewed papers, the monograph *Breastfeeding in hospital: Mothers, midwives and the production line* (2006), and joint editor of books including *Infant and young child* *feeding: Challenges to implementing a global strategy* (2009) and *Ethnographic research in maternal and child health* (2016).

Francesca Entwistle is a midwife of over 30 years and works as Professional Officer (policy and advocacy) at Unicef UK Baby Friendly Initiative. Her specialist interest in breastfeeding was consolidated through her research exploring the impact of midwifery training and women's self-efficacy on breastfeeding outcomes for women from low-income groups. She has worked with the UK Department of Health in developing policy and practice in relation to maternal and infant nutrition, and regularly consults with key stakeholders, to ensure the focus on improving public health through breastfeeding and very early child development in the UK continues. Francesca leads the National Infant Feeding Network and is a visiting lecturer at the University of Hertfordshire.

Melanie Fraser is a Visiting Fellow of the Centre for Public Health and Wellbeing of the University of the West of England, Bristol. She has both worked and studied in the Faculties of Health and Applied Sciences and Business and Law. The chapter in this volume is drawn from her doctoral work. She taught law for many years and has an LLB and a master's degree in employment law. She is a qualified Breastfeeding Counsellor with the Association of Breastfeeding Mothers, and is the mother of two breastfed children.

Fiona Giles teaches in Media and Communications at Sydney University. She has published in breastfeeding studies for over twenty years, and is the author of *Fresh milk: The secret life of breasts* (2003) and numerous scholarly articles on the experiential and cultural meanings of breastfeeding. Recent publications include 'Towards social maternity: where's the mother? Stories from a transgender dad as a case study of human milk sharing', in *Bioethics beyond altruism: Donating and transforming biological materials* (2017).

Sally Johnson has worked in public health for 17 years and completed her MSc Public Health in 2013. She currently leads on maternal and early years public health for Wiltshire Council. Her portfolio includes leading on the local breastfeeding strategy and commissioning services that support women to breastfeed. She works closely with maternity, health visiting and children's centre services, among others, and is passionate about improving integrated care for women and families from conception to five years.

Emma Laird is an Early Years Practitioner who works in a Bristol Children's Centre. She is committed to supporting women to breastfeed and for over eight years has supported mothers to breastfeed in a weekly group.

Dawn Leeming is a Principal Lecturer in Psychology and Director of Graduate Education for the School of Human and Health Sciences at the University of Huddersfield. Previously she worked within NHS mental health services as a clinical psychologist. She has researched several aspects of health and wellbeing, with a particular interest in the psychology of emotion, the impact on wellbeing of service user understandings of psychological distress and mental health stigma, and women's wellbeing in relation to infant feeding and transition to motherhood. She has a particular interest in the emotional aspects of breastfeeding support.

Abigail Locke is a critical social psychologist whose research work has a discursive flavour. She investigates topics around gender, parenting, identity and health. She has an interest in what society constructs as 'good' mothering and fathering, and has examined topics around infant feeding, birthing experiences and stay-at-home fathers. A particular focus is on the advice that is given to new parents. Abigail is currently Professor of Psychology at the University of Bradford, and Visiting Professor in Social and Health Psychology at the University of Derby.

Geraldine Lucas trained as a nurse and spent eight years in the Royal Navy working in a variety of settings before training as a midwife. In 2004 she joined the University of the West of England, Bristol, as a midwifery lecturer. Her midwifery experience in practice included working with a small team of midwives to provide one-to-one care for women who experienced or developed complications during their pregnancy. She has a range of teaching interests, including interprofessional simulation with midwifery and medical students, breastfeeding and sustainability. Geraldine is passionate about the integration of breastfeeding education, the quality of student learning and the mirroring of this learning within practice to support breastfeeding mothers.

Elizabeth Mayo is an NCT Breastfeeding Counsellor, Tutor and Assessor who attends a breastfeeding group each week. She trains peer supporters to work in a person-centred model to support the parents at the group.

Lucila Newell holds a PhD in geography from the Open University. Her research focuses on the weaving of socio-natural relations in different spaces and around different issues, from work on socio-natures in cities and the politics of waste, to breastfeeding and the connection with nature. She is currently an Associate Researcher in the Centre for Cultures of Reproduction, Technologies and Health (CORTH) and the Centre for Global Health Policy in the School of Global Studies, at the University of Sussex. She has trained and volunteered as a breastfeeding peer supporter for more than a year and is co-founder of a social enterprise called The Parlour, which aims at creating a space for mothers who breastfeed, to share stories, explore the issues surrounding breastfeeding and generate new images of breastfeeding mothers.

David Pontin holds the Aneurin Bevan Chair of Community Health, Faculty of Life Sciences and Education, University of South Wales, UK. He is a registered nurse (for adults and children) and a health visitor/public health nurse, and teaches postgraduate students on the Public Health, Advanced Clinical Practice, and Specialist Community Public Health Nursing programmes, as well as supervising postgraduate research students. He is co-chair of the FLSE Community Health and Care Cognate Group, as well as a member of MetaPH, which explores complexity theory and public health (www.metaPH.org), and Holi, an evaluation group linked with Co-production Wales (https://copronet. wales). David's current research focuses on family resilience (www.frait. wales) and the implications for health visiting practice. His interest in breastfeeding stems from his clinical practice as a nurse/health visitor, and his experience as a father.

Lisa Smyth is a Senior Lecturer in Sociology at Queen's University Belfast. Her research interests centre on social roles and interaction, with a focus on gender, reproduction and family life. She is currently working on a monograph titled *Roles, conflict and anxiety*. She has previously published *The demands of motherhood: Agents, roles and recognition* (2012) and *Abortion and nation: The politics of reproduction in contemporary Ireland* (2005).

Nicki Symes is a nurse, midwife and health visitor who has an interest in improving women's health and raising breastfeeding rates. She currently works as a Public Health Principal in Maternal and Infant Health at Bristol City Council.

Sally Tedstone is currently an infant feeding specialist working in maternity services. She has been a midwife for over 25 years, and has a first degree in adult education and an MSc in public health. Sally has worked in infant feeding since around 2000 in a number of roles, including Senior Professional Officer for Unicef UK Baby Friendly Initiative, Infant Feeding and Healthy Early Years Lead for the Department of Health, and Infant Feeding Lead for Wales.

Cecilia Tomori is Assistant Professor of Anthropology and member of the Parent–Infant Sleep Lab at Durham University. She is the author of *Nighttime breastfeeding: An American cultural dilemma* (2014) and co-editor of *Breastfeeding: New anthropological approaches* (2017). Her research focuses on the dynamic interaction of the sociocultural and biological aspects of breastfeeding and infant sleep.

Acknowledgements

There are very many people that we need to say thank you to for their help and support in both running the seminar series and in bringing the book together. We are very grateful to the Economic and Social Research Council (ESRC) for funding the seminar series. Others include, in no particular order:

- The conference support teams from the various venues: UWE, Bristol; Cardiff University; the National Museum Wales; and Watershed, Bristol;
- For help with booking, organising the events and keeping the website tidy, a big thank you to the post-award support team at UWE, Bristol;
- All the people who came to the seminars, either as presenters or attendees, and their colleagues for holding the fort while they were away.

And finally, we want to thank all of the people who support breastfeeding women wherever they may be.

Introduction

Sally Dowling, David Pontin and Kate Boyer

Background

This book seeks to draw together lessons learned from a recent series of seminars held in the UK, focused on breastfeeding. We faced many challenges as editors: How could we represent and do justice to something that was lively, dynamic, exciting and changeable, for a person who wasn't there? How could we make sure that the essence of what we thought the thing was about is present, recognisable to those who attended and intelligible to those who weren't there for all or part of the time? These are some of the questions that we wrestled with when we started to sketch out our ideas for the structure, form and content of this book.

As the title of the book suggests, the overarching focus of the seminars was breastfeeding research, policy and practice. The seminars were hosted by three UK universities: the University of the West of England, Bristol (UWE); Cardiff University; and the University of South Wales (USW). They took place during 2015 and 2016, with the location rotating between Cardiff and Bristol.

The 'thing' was a series of six, day-long seminars, supported and funded by the UK Economic and Social Research Council (ESRC). Sally Dowling (UWE), Kate Boyer (Cardiff University), David Pontin (USW) and Julie Mytton (UWE) applied for support for the seminar series in 2014, as it addressed the ESRC's strategic priority of 'Influencing behaviour and informing interventions', and particularly the research topics of 'understanding behaviour', 'social diversity' and 'health and wellbeing'. There are few spaces where people from different backgrounds can meet, talk, listen and consider breastfeeding from differing but complementary perspectives, and where they can collaborate in knowledge creation. Other UK fora exist for discussing research in relation to policy and practice – the Unicef UK Baby Friendly Initiative Annual Conference is a good example. For highlighting research from a range of disciplines there is the biennial UK Maternal and Infant Nutrition and Nurture Conference. However, none of these highlights the relationships between theory, policy and practice, and collaborative knowledge-making, in the way that we set out to do. We wanted to use the seminars to facilitate a series of conversations about current issues in breastfeeding, and to synthesise new knowledge. This book is a physical artefact that has come out of the series, and other projects are afoot –publications in peer-reviewed and practitioner-focused journals, and grant bidding activities.

We wanted to create a space where people could meet to consider how to further our understanding of women's embodied, affective and day-to-day experiences of trying to breastfeed their babies, and to talk about how more UK women might be helped to breastfeed their babies for longer. The speakers were chosen for the relevance and originality of their breastfeeding work, and while the UK-specific policy context was the starting point for the seminar series, we recognise that the issues we talked about have wider relevance and influences. We planned to have about thirty participants at each seminar, including speakers with international and interdisciplinary representation to promote a wide perspective, and to create opportunities for synergies, knowledge transfer and collaborative problem-solving. Our aim was to have speakers and participants from every level – from early career researchers to international experts, practitioners and policy makers (governmental and nongovernmental). A core group of UK academics, policy makers and practitioners was invited to attend all six seminars to develop a strand of ongoing conversations between the seminars and across the series, so that we didn't keep starting from the beginning each time. Additional seminar places were made available for local practitioners such as infant feeding coordinators, breastfeeding peer supporters and representatives from voluntary organisations. Most places were free; others were offered at minimal cost. Twelve free places were offered to PhD students/early career researchers during the series to help them maximise their networking and to support future researchers.

Breastfeeding in the UK

Breastfeeding is a policy priority for the four devolved UK governments with a responsibility for health (England DH, 2009; Northern Ireland DHSSP, 2013; Welsh Government, 2016; Scottish Government, 2017), and is acknowledged to be important in improving public health and reducing health inequalities (WHO, 2017). This is supported by good quality evidence which was updated and further reinforced by the *Lancet* series of papers which were published during the seminar series lifetime (see Rollins et al, 2016; Victora et al, 2016). Although UK breastfeeding initiation rates are typically high, they fall rapidly: data from the last Infant Feeding Survey suggests that only 55% of women breastfeed their babies at six weeks, 34% are still breastfeeding their babies at six months, with most women who give up breastfeeding early expressing regret at their decision (McAndrew et al, 2012). Recent figures published during the preparation of this volume indicate that a third of women stop breastfeeding by six weeks (ISD Scotland, 2016; PHE 2017a), and the Unicef call to action (2016) and the recent Cochrane Review (McFadden et al, 2017) emphasise the importance of social and cultural support for breastfeeding.

There is a clear relationship in the UK between socioeconomic status and breastfeeding, with significantly lower rates among women living in the most deprived areas. There are also differences between younger mothers and older mothers, women with different levels of formal education, and women from different ethnic backgrounds (McAndrew et al, 2012). This is seen in the local data for the Department of Health (DH) (PHE, 2017b). Reducing inequalities by increasing breastfeeding rates is recognised in policy, and 'breastfeeding initiation' and 'breastfeeding at 6–8 weeks' are health improvement indicators in the Public Health Outcomes Framework (DH, 2017). There is also a growing body of evidence supporting the economic reasons for encouraging more mothers to initiate and sustain breastfeeding. For just five illnesses, for example, a moderate increase in the number of mothers breastfeeding for the minimum advised period translates into cost savings for the UK NHS of £40 million (Renfrew et al, 2012; Pokhrel et al, 2015).

At first glance the breastfeeding of babies appears to be straightforward – with the common belief that it's a natural thing and therefore easy to do. However, on closer examination it quickly shows itself to be a complex, 'wicked' social problem (Braithwaite et al, 2017). 'Wicked' because the reasons for variation in breastfeeding rates are complicated and multifaceted, and include social and cultural factors such as type and level of support available to pregnant women and breastfeeding mothers. Interventions at different levels, from individual interactions between mothers and their peers to governmental and global health policy, are important in promoting meaningful changes to support mothers in breastfeeding (Labbok et al 2008). Although UK initiation rates suggest that the 'breast is best' message is being acknowledged and absorbed (in some areas by some mothers), the breastfeeding duration rates remain variable (NHS Digital, 2012: 16).

The variation in available breastfeeding support is part of the story, as is the loss of intergenerational kin-based knowledge networks. In addition, a whole range of micro-practices, social engagements and events unfold when mothers try to integrate breastfeeding into the rest of their lives. It is these parts of the story that the seminar series focused on – the nuances of breastfeeding babies as a social practice. We wanted to shed some light on why some mothers breastfeed and some do not, and why some stop when they do.

Aims of the seminar series

We wanted to try and answer the following questions:

- How does attending to the micro-practices and affective and embodied experiences of breastfeeding women advance extant knowledge about the reasons for breastfeeding cessation?
- How can we further our understanding about inequalities in breastfeeding rates by focusing on the nuances of day-to-day breastfeeding?
- How might an increased understanding of these perspectives influence policy?

In editing the book, we wanted to make sure that all voices had the opportunity to be heard. So, when we were planning the book structure, we invited practitioners/policy makers to provide commentaries on the different sections of the book. The chapters are based on some of the presentations from the seminars (see Appendix for details), and give a flavour of the dialogue that we facilitated. Not all presenters were in a position to contribute a chapter to the book – Dr Kate Boyer, Cardiff University; Dr Danielle Groleau, McGill University, Canada; April Whincop, Barnardo's Breastfeeding Peer Support Co-ordinator, Bristol; Dr Catherine Angell, University of Bournemouth; and Dr Shantini Paranjothy, Cardiff University, were unable to contribute – and the absence of their work is no indication of the quality of presentations or their reception on the day. If you want to find out more about what went on then please visit the seminar series website, where you'll find edited audio files of the presentations and background information.

During seminar series planning we drew on our experience of similar events. Sally and David have attended the Breastfeeding and Feminism International Conference series (there is more on this connection in the Conclusion) and Kate took part in the ESRC seminar series 'Feminism and futurity: new times, new spaces' (2009–10). We noted that the number of presentations in that seminar series, the presentation–discussion ratio and breakout sessions allowed participants time to discuss ideas in depth and establish continuing networks. In a bid to share the model with others who might be considering such an event, we provide a short overview here, and we are very happy to share our experience in more detail.

A typical breastfeeding seminar series session started with an informal gathering for some networking. We wanted people to be relaxed and to make new connections so they felt comfortable to share their experience and contribute to new knowledge production. Once the session started, a more organised series of introductions followed, whereby all the people attending introduced themselves and said where they were from. For every session, the room was organised cafe style, with approximately 6–8 people per 'home' table, and there were usually 30–40 people per session – the core group, presenters, and local practitioners and policy makers. We purposefully arranged the seating plan to ensure that each table had a mixture of practitioners, policy makers and academics, so that no one voice was dominant, to encourage a meaningful dialogue between the different perspectives. We were mindful that this might be different from what people were used to, and Sally Tedstone has written an evaluation piece (see 'Seminar series context') based on people's experiences of attending.

The morning session typically featured two presentations, usually delivered by one international and one UK academic. Each presentation was followed by a brief questions and answers session for clarifying information. Before lunch, each home table discussed what they had heard, so everyone could speak about their experience and understandings. We then facilitated a whole-room review, where each table shared key points and issues for consideration. The pattern repeated after lunch with another academic presentation and a policy/practice presentation, followed by a final panel discussion of issues raised by the attendees. For the last seminar, chaired by Dr Julie Mytton, we reserved the afternoon for presentations from PhD students and early career researchers (Gretel Finch, Bristol University; Laura Streeter, London School of Hygiene and Tropical Medicine; Lula Mecinska, Lancaster University; and Sharon Tugwell, Birkbeck, University of London) so that they could share their work with a diverse audience. The series concluded on a celebratory note and featured a performance by UK spoken-word artist Hollie McNish. Her powerful piece on YouTube about breastfeeding in public has been seen nearly 1.5 million times and you can access it online to get a flavour of her presentation, which also drew on her book *Nobody told me* (2017).

Developments during the series

The seminar series straddled a two-year period, during which there were some interesting UK breastfeeding developments. In 2014, the highly regarded Infant Feeding Survey was stood down, and there were major changes in collecting and collating official breastfeeding data (NHS Digital, 2014). The Westminster Parliament All-Party Parliamentary Group on Infant Feeding and Inequalities was formed in 2016 (WBTI, 2017) and members of the core team were invited to their inaugural meeting; others have also attended subsequently. During 2017 Alison Thewliss MP asked questions about breastfeeding in the House of Commons, started a campaign to encourage Scottish football grounds to become 'breastfeeding friendly', published a bill on infant formula promotion and launched an inquiry into infant feeding policy (which was unfortunately interrupted by the 2017 General Election).

The *Lancet* also published a breastfeeding series in which updated systematic reviews of evidence were used to highlight issues with breastfeeding rates and cultural support for breastfeeding (Rollins et al, 2016; Victora et al, 2016). The accompanying editorial urged governments and health authorities to work together to 'establish a new normal: where every woman can expect to breastfeed, and to receive every support she needs to do so' (*Lancet*, 2016: 404). This was closely followed by an 'Open letter on the UK breastfeeding crisis' and signatories included contributors to this volume and seminar attendees. The Unicef Call to Action on Breastfeeding was launched in 2016 (Unicef, 2016), as was the World Breastfeeding Trends Initiative UK report (2016) (WBTI, 2017). Some of this dynamism is reflected in the chapters and we hope that they inspire academics, policy makers and practitioners to continue promoting breastfeeding.

Structure of the book

Following this introduction, we include a 'UK policy context' piece by Francesca Entwistle and Fiona Dykes. They draw on their joint presentation at the final seminar of the series to talk about the Unicef UK Baby Friendly Initiative reconfiguration to reflect the importance of relationships and ensure sustainability. The remainder of the book is divided into three sections: I) Breastfeeding and emotions, II) Cultures of breastfeeding, and III) Breastfeeding and popular culture. Each section contains four loosely related chapters, based on the authors' presentations during the seminar series. The relationships between chapters both within and between sections are discussed further in the Conclusion. A 'Commentary' follows each group of chapters, written by pairs or groups of core seminar participants working in breastfeeding policy/practice roles. We asked commentary writers to write in whatever form they thought appropriate: we have a reflective conversation (in Part I), a more traditional piece (Part II) and a reflection on learning, including quotes from the authors (Part III). Finally, a 'Seminar series context' piece by Sally Tedstone reflects on the experience of attending the seminar series from different perspectives. A conclusion draws the book's themes together and considers these in relation to our aims for the series.

Terminology

Finally, we need to say something about our decision to use the phrase 'infant formula'. We experimented with different, technically correct terms – for example, 'artificial breast-milk substitute' – but this made the various texts ungainly and difficult to read. So, we take our lead from the First Steps Nutrition 2017 report on infant milks in the UK:

> We use the term infant formula to mean a food that can meet all an infant's nutritional needs during the first six months of life and alongside complementary food for the second six months, and which complies with the regulations for infant formula. (Crawley and Westland, 2017: section 2:2)

We hope this does not obscure the meaning of the messages contained within, that you enjoy reading the chapters and commentaries, and that the book gives you something of the flavour of the events.

References

Braithwaite, J., Churruca, K., Ellis, L. A., Long, J., Clay-Williams, R., Damen, N., Herkes, J., Pomare, C. and Ludlow K. (2017) 'Complexity science in healthcare: Aspirations, approaches, applications and accomplishments: a white paper', Sydney: Australian Institute of Health Innovation, Macquarie University, www.hsraanz. org/wp-content/uploads/Braithwaite-2017-Complexity-Science-in-Healthcare-A-White-Paper.pdf

Crawley, H. and Westland, S. (2017) 'Infant milks in the UK: A practical guide for health professionals', http://firststepsnutrition.org/pdfs/Infant_Milks_July2017.pdf

Department of Health (2009) 'Healthy child programme: Pregnancy and the first five years of life', London: DH, https://www.gov.uk/government/uploads/system/uploads/attachment_data/file/167998/Health_Child_Programme.pdf

Department of Health (2017) 'Public Health Outcomes Framework', London: DH, http://fingertipsreports.phe.org.uk/public-health-outcomes-framework/e06000025.pdf

Department of Health, Social Services and Public Safety (2013) 'Breastfeeding: A great start: A strategy for Northern Ireland 2013 –2023', Belfast: DHSSPS, www.health-ni.gov.uk/sites/default/files/publications/dhssps/breastfeeding-strategy-2014.pdf

Information Services Division Scotland (2017) 'Breastfeeding statistics: Financial year 2015/16', https://www.isdscotland.org/Health-Topics/Child-Health/Publications/2016-10-25/2016-10-25-Breastfeeding-Report.pdf

Labbok, M. H., Hall Smith, P. and Taylor, E. C. (2008) 'Breastfeeding and feminism: a focus on reproductive health, rights and justice', *International Breastfeeding Journal*, 3: 8.

Lancet (2016) 'Editorial: breastfeeding: achieving the new normal', *Lancet*, 376: 404.

McAndrew, F., Thompson, J., Fellows, L., Large, A., Speed, M. and Renfrew, M. J. (2012) 'Infant feeding survey: 2010', NHS Information Centre, http://data.gov.uk/dataset/infant-feeding-survey-2010

McFadden, A., Gavine, A., Renfrew, M. J., Wade, A., Buchanan, P., Taylor, J. L., Veitch, E., Rennie, A. M., Crowther, S. A., Neiman, S. and MacGillivray, S. (2017) 'Support for healthy breastfeeding mothers with healthy term babies', *Cochrane Database of Systematic Reviews*, 2, art. no.: CD001141.

McNish, H. (2017) *Nobody told me: poetry and parenthood*, London: Blackfriars.

NHS Digital (2012) 'Chapter 2: Incidence, prevalence and duration of breastfeeding', *Infant Feeding Survey – UK, 2010*, http://content.digital.nhs.uk/catalogue/PUB08694/ifs-uk-2010-chap2-inc-prev-dur.pdf

NHS Digital (2014) 'The infant feeding survey has been discontinued', http://content.digital.nhs.uk/media/20585/IFS-Notice/pdf/IFSNotice.pdf

Pokhrel, S., Quigley, M. A., Fox-Rushby, J., McCormick, F., Williams, A., Trueman, P., Dodds, R. and Renfrew M. J. (2015) 'Potential economic impacts from improving breastfeeding rates in the UK', *Archives of Disease in Childhood*, 100: 334–40, http://adc.bmj.com/content/100/4/334.long

Public Health England (2017a) 'Breastfeeding at 6 to 8 weeks after birth: 2016 to 2017 quarterly data', https://www.gov.uk/government/statistics/breastfeeding-at-6-to-8-weeks-after-birth-2016-to-2017-quarterly-data

Public Health England (2017b) 'Guidance: Child and maternal health data and intelligence: a guide for health professionals', https://www.gov.uk/guidance/child-and-maternal-health-data-and-intelligence-a-guide-for-health-professionals

Renfrew, M. J., Pokhrel, S., Quigley, M., McCormick, F., Fox-Rushby, J., Dodds, R., Duffy, S., Trueman, P. and Williams, A. (2012) 'Preventing disease and saving resources: The potential contribution of increasing breastfeeding rates in the UK', www.unicef.org.uk/Documents/Baby_Friendly/Research/Preventing_disease_saving_resources.pdf

Rollins, N. C., Bhandari, N., Hajeebhoy, N., Horton, S., Lutter, C. K., Martines, J. C., Piwoz, E. G., Richter, L. M. and Victora, C. G., on behalf of the Lancet Breastfeeding Series Group (2016) 'Why invest, and what it will take to improve breastfeeding practices?', *The Lancet*, 387(10017): 491–504.

Scottish Government (2017) *Best start: A five-year forward plan for maternity and neonatal care in Scotland*, Edinburgh: Scottish Government, https://beta.gov.scot/publications/best-start-five-year-forward-plan-maternity-neonatal-care-scotland

Unicef (2016) 'Protecting health and saving lives: A call to action, Unicef UK Baby Friendly Initiative', https://www.unicef.org.uk/babyfriendly/wp-content/uploads/sites/2/2016/04/Call-to-Action-Unicef-UK-Baby-Friendly-Initiative.pdf

Victora, C. G., Bahl, R., Barros, A.J.D., França, G.V.A., Horton, S., Krasevec, J., Murch, S., Sankar, M. J., Walker, N. and Rollins N. C., for the Lancet Breastfeeding Series Group (2016) 'Breastfeeding in the 21st century: epidemiology, mechanisms, and lifelong effect', *The Lancet*, 387 (10017): 475–90.

Welsh Government (2016) 'An overview of the Healthy Child Wales Programme', Cardiff: Welsh Government, http://gov.wales/topics/health/publications/health/reports/healthy-child/?lang=en

WHO (2017) 'Infant and young child feeding fact sheet', Geneva: WHO, www.who.int/mediacentre/factsheets/fs342/en

World Breastfeeding Trends Initiative (2016) 'UK report 2016', https://ukbreastfeeding.org/wbtiuk2016

The UK policy context: reconfiguration of the Unicef UK Baby Friendly Initiative to reflect the importance of relationships and ensuring sustainability

Francesca Entwistle and Fiona Dykes

Introduction

Over the last 20 years, the Unicef UK Baby Friendly Initiative (BFI) has succeeded in gaining national recognition for the importance of breastfeeding and creating new 'common knowledge' related to many breastfeeding practices in the health service and among policy makers. For example, once hotly debated topics such as skin-to-skin contact, rooming in, teaching mothers how to breastfeed and avoiding supplements are now accepted as good practice. While not every mother in the UK receives this level of support, overall standards have improved and breastfeeding initiation rates have steadily increased: from 62% in 1990, to 76% in 2005, to 81% in 2010 (McAndrew et al, 2012), with 84% of all infants now born into a Baby Friendly accredited hospital (Unicef UK, 2017a).

Despite this progress, as well as the overwhelming evidence that breastfeeding saves lives, improves health and cuts costs, breastfeeding continuation rates in the UK remain some of the lowest in the world (Victora et al, 2016). Infant formula feeding is entrenched in society as the cultural norm (Unicef UK, 2016a); the physiological norm of breastfeeding, with the concurrent emotional attachment and relationship-building, has been interrupted. Having raised the foundation level of knowledge and skills within maternity care in the UK, in 2012 the Unicef UK BFI incorporated new evidence and developed additional Baby Friendly standards, including a focus on supporting parents to build close and loving relationships with their infants (Unicef UK, 2013). Building on the success of the BFI, the new standards aim to further improve the health and wellbeing outcomes for all infants and their mothers, irrespective of their feeding method.

Historical overview

In 1989, to reverse the alarming global trend towards increased use of breast milk substitutes and to raise the momentum of political pressure on infant formula companies to stop undermining breastfeeding, the World Health Organization (WHO) and Unicef published a joint statement: *Protecting, promoting and supporting breastfeeding* (WHO/ Unicef, 1989). This statement included 'Ten steps to successful breastfeeding' (see Figure 1).

Figure 1: 10 steps to successful breastfeeding

Every facility providing maternity services and care for newborn infants should...
1. Have a written breastfeeding policy that is routinely communicated to all healthcare staff
2. Train all healthcare staff in the skills necessary to implement the breastfeeding policy
3. Inform all pregnant women about the benefits and management of breastfeeding
4. Help mothers to initiate breastfeeding within half an hour of birth
5. Show mothers how to breastfeed and how to maintain lactation even if they are separated from their infants
6. Give newborn infants no food or drink other than breast milk, unless medically indicated
7. Practice rooming-in, allowing mothers and infants to remain together 24 hours a day
8. Encourage breastfeeding on demand
9. Give no artificial teats or pacifiers (also called dummies or soothers) to breastfeeding infants
10. Foster the establishment of breastfeeding support groups and refer mothers to them on discharge from the hospital or clinic

Source: WHO/Unicef (1989)

In 1991, WHO/Unicef launched the global Baby Friendly Hospital Initiative (BFHI). The purpose of this initiative was to support the development of an infrastructure in maternity care facilities that enabled them to implement the Ten Steps (WHO/Unicef, 1992). National teams were set up in participating countries, with the remit of coordinating and monitoring implementation in hospitals. A Baby Friendly Award would be issued to those facilities that reached a minimum externally auditable standard in relation to the Ten Steps. The BFHI was adopted in the UK in 1994 and was renamed the Unicef UK Baby Friendly Initiative (BFI) to emphasise that it was not solely related to hospitals, with an adapted programme being developed for community facilities in 1998.

The global BFHI sought to reverse harmful infant feeding and related practices through the removal of constraints to breastfeeding, such as clinical routines, hospital nurseries and advertising of breast milk substitutes, along with improved education of staff. This global script was particularly appealing in the face of the devastation that the introduction of Western medical dogma and commercial activity had upon women's birthing and breastfeeding experiences in countries around the world. Inhumane norms had developed, such as women labouring and birthing in a supine position on uncovered metal trolleys, with their babies being forcibly extracted and separated to a stark nursery and fed breast milk substitutes (Dykes, 2006). Equally devastating were the effects of poverty and lack of access to clean water upon the lives of babies and families when women used breast milk substitutes (Dykes, 2006).

The mode of implementation of the BFHI involved what Wright (1998) describes as a deliberate unsettling and replacing of a dominant ideology, requiring not just political activity but interventions in 'culture', involving manipulation of words, renaming and redefining key concepts. However, a major challenge, as with other global strategies, stems from the attempt to make uniform changes across the globe in enormously diverse cultural settings (Dykes and Hall Moran, 2009).

Over twenty years later, the BFHI has expanded across the globe (WHO, 2017). A recent systematic review identified that implementation of the BFHI has a positive impact on short-, medium- and long-term breastfeeding outcomes, with a dose–response relationship between the number of BFHI steps women are exposed to and the likelihood of improved breastfeeding outcomes (Pérez-Escamilla et al, 2016). However, despite this success, criticisms have been levied related to the BFHI being baby- rather than mother-friendly (Schmied et al, 2014).

Responding to the evidence: Unicef UK Baby Friendly standards 2012

In the UK, a more nuanced BFI approach has been developed based on evidence regarding women's preferences for person-centred approaches (Schmied et al, 2011) and the importance of prioritising relationships, to better facilitate mothers' capacities to respond to their babies' cues (Dykes and Flacking, 2010; Thomson et al, 2012). To facilitate this paradigm shift, Unicef UK produced a set of evidence-based revised standards for maternity, neonatal, health visiting and children's centre services (Unicef UK, 2012). These standards are more holistic, child rights-based and consistent with developmental science evidence for very early child development (Shonkoff and Garner, 2012), focusing on feeding and relationship-building for all babies, mothers and their families, irrespective of infant feeding method. These new messages within the BFI standards and guidance form part of a comprehensive approach to supporting parents in raising healthy, prosocial children.

Between 2012 and 2017, the Unicef UK BFI supported a transition for health services to implement the new Baby Friendly standards (Unicef UK, 2016b). This approach ensured that the momentum for implementing BFI in the UK continued to support an established infrastructure of infant feeding, building on the Baby Friendly process of 'standards, assessment and accreditation', while also incorporating the new standards around helping parents to build a close and loving relationship with their infant from pregnancy into the early postnatal period. Currently, there is no formal evaluation of the new standards; however, anecdotal evidence from Infant Feeding leads and Baby Friendly assessors is that the standards have been well received, staff feel that they are 'just right' and they are helping to embed a growing body of evidence on what works to further support very early child development (APPG for Conception to Age 2, 2014). The new standards value breastfeeding not only as a means of providing food, but as a way for the baby and mother to become securely attached, encouraging the mother to be responsive to her baby's needs not only for food, but for love, comfort and protection. In addition, the standards support infant formula-feeding mothers to be responsive to their babies' needs and to build close and loving relationships with them (see Table 1).

Table 1: The Unicef UK revised Baby Friendly standards (2012)

Maternity	Neonatal	Health visiting	Children centres
1. Support pregnant women to recognise the importance of breastfeeding and early relationships for the health and wellbeing of their baby	1. Support parents to have a close and loving relationship with their baby	1. Support pregnant women to recognise the importance of breastfeeding and early relationships for the health and wellbeing of their baby	1. Support pregnant women to recognise the importance of breastfeeding and early relationships for the health and wellbeing of their baby
2. Support all mothers and babies to initiate a close and loving relationship and feeding soon after birth	2. Enable babies to receive breast milk and to breastfeed when possible	2. Enable mothers to continue to breastfeed for as long as they wish	2. Protect and support breastfeeding in all areas of the service
3. Enable mothers to get breastfeeding off to a good start	3. Value parents as partners in care	3. Support mothers to make informed decisions regarding the introduction of food or fluids other than breast milk	3. Support parents to have a close and loving relationship with their baby
4. Support mothers to make informed decisions regarding the introduction of food or fluids other than breast milk		4. Support parents to have a close and loving relationship with their baby	
5. Support parents to have a close and loving relationship with their baby			

Achieving sustainability

A strong theme emerging from the review process was that the Baby Friendly standards are hard to maintain in the long term. It was therefore decided that achieving sustainability should be part of the new Baby Friendly standards from the beginning, and a new award should be introduced to encourage focus on sustainability after the initial accreditation: Baby Friendly Accreditation with Sustainability (Gold Award).

A service is achieving sustainability when it has implemented and maintained the core Baby Friendly standards, confirmed by a full reassessment. In addition, they must have adequate leadership structures in place to support continued maintenance and evaluation of the standards and for progressing and improving the standards over time.

The service must also demonstrate that it cultivates a positive and enabling culture for Baby Friendly, which considers the specific cultural and societal challenges in the UK (Unicef UK, 2016c) (see Table 2).

Table 2 The Achieving Sustainability standards (2016)

Leadership	Culture	Monitoring	Progression
Develop a leadership team that promotes the Baby Friendly standards	Foster an organisational culture that protects the Baby Friendly standards	Construct robust monitoring processes to support the Baby Friendly standards	Continue to develop the service in order to sustain the Baby Friendly standards

What happens after services have achieved sustainability?

In 2017, Unicef UK BFI accredited the first two services (one maternity and one community) with a 'Gold Award', Achieving Sustainability. It is envisaged that these services that are sustaining the core Baby Friendly standards now have the systems, leadership, culture and audit in place to help them continue to promote, protect and support breastfeeding, and to support all mothers to build a close and loving relationship with their baby.

Once accredited, the service is expected to keep a portfolio to record successes and challenges relating to all the standards, including evidence of action planning and evaluation. This portfolio will be submitted annually to Unicef UK. One year after the initial Gold accreditation, a meeting will take place with a Unicef UK Baby Friendly assessor to review the portfolio and review the action taken to address any recommendations made during the reassessment visit and/or Achieving Sustainability assessment. Following this meeting, further formal revalidation meetings will take place with a Baby Friendly assessor every three years. Short-notice monitoring visits will be carried out by Unicef UK on a percentage of facilities holding a Gold Award every year.

Conclusion

The Baby Friendly Initiative is improving breastfeeding rates and practice to support breastfeeding, but maintaining these positive results requires continued resourcing as well as interventions beyond the healthcare context (Unicef UK, 2017b). In 2016, Unicef UK launched a Call to Action campaign urging UK governments to take steps to support and promote breastfeeding, and to protect all babies from commercial interests; this included recommendations that all UK babies should be born in a Baby Friendly hospital to ensure that their mothers have the best possible opportunity to get breastfeeding off to a good start (Unicef UK, 2016a). However, the UK's low breastfeeding rates are not the responsibility of individual women (Rollins et al, 2016), but of society as a whole. Full implementation and sustainability of the Unicef UK Baby Friendly standards provides a firm foundation for breastfeeding success. The next step is for everyone in society to come together to remove the practical, emotional and cultural barriers to breastfeeding, as well as to create an enabling environment for all women who want to breastfeed, and for breastfeeding to once again be seen as the 'normal' way to feed and nurture a baby.

References

All Parliamentary Party Group (APPG) for Conception to Age 2: First 1001 Days (2014) 'The 1001 Critical Days: The importance of the conception to age two period', http://www.1001criticaldays.co.uk/home

Dykes, F. (2006) *Breastfeeding in hospital: Mothers, midwives and the production line*, London: Routledge.

Dykes, F. and Flacking, R. (2010) 'Encouraging breastfeeding: a relational perspective', *Early Human Development*, 86: 733–6.

Dykes, F. and Hall Moran, V. (2009) (eds) *Infant and young child feeding: Challenges to implementing a global strategy*, Oxford: Wiley-Blackwell.

McAndrew, F., Thompson, J., Fellows, L., Large, A., Speed, M. and Renfrew, M. J. (2012) 'Infant Feeding Survey 2010', London: Health and Social Care Information Centre, http://content.digital.nhs.uk/catalogue/PUB08694/Infant-Feeding-Survey-2010-Consolidated-Report.pdf

Pérez-Escamilla, R., Martinez, J. L. and Segura-Pérez, S. (2016) 'Impact of the Baby-friendly Hospital Initiative on breastfeeding and child health outcomes: a systematic review', *Maternal and Child Nutrition*, 12 (3): 402–17.

Rollins, N. C., Bhandari, N., Hajeebhoy, N., Horton, S., Lutter, C. K., Martines, J. C., Piwoz, E. G., Richter, L. M. and Victora C. G. on behalf of The Lancet Breastfeeding Series Group (2016) 'Why invest, and what it will take to improve breastfeeding practices?', *Lancet*, 387(10017): 491–504.

Schmied, V., Beake, S., Sheehan, A., McCourt, C. and Dykes, F. (2011) 'Women's perceptions and experiences of breastfeeding support: a metasynthesis', *Birth: Issues in Perinatal Care*, 38: 49–60.

Schmied, V., Thomson, G., Sheehan, A., Burns, E., Byrom, A. and Dykes, F. (2014) 'A meta-ethnographic study of health care staff perceptions of the WHO/Unicef Baby Friendly Health Initiative', *Women and Birth*, 27: 242–9.

Shonkoff, J. P., Garner, A. S., Committee on Psychosocial Aspects of Child and Family Health; Committee on Early Childhood, Adoption, and Dependent Care; and Section on Developmental and Behavioral Pediatrics (2012) 'The lifelong effects of early childhood adversity and toxic stress', *Pediatrics*, 129: e232–e246.

Thomson, G., Bilson, A. and Dykes, F. (2012) '"Changing hearts and minds": An evaluation of implementation of Unicef UK Baby Friendly Initiative in the community', *Midwifery*, 28: 258–64.

Unicef UK (2012) Guide to the Baby Friendly Initiative Standards, https://www.unicef.org.uk/babyfriendly/baby-friendly-resources/guidance-for-health-professionals/implementing-the-baby-friendly-standards/guide-to-the-baby-friendly-initiative-standards/

Unicef UK (2013) Evidence and rationale for the Unicef UK Baby Friendly Initiative Standards, https://www.unicef.org.uk/babyfriendly/baby-friendly-resources/advocacy/the-evidence-and-rationale-for-the-unicef-uk-baby-friendly-initiative-standards/

Unicef UK (2016a) Protecting health and saving lives: A call to action, https://www.unicef.org.uk/babyfriendly/wp-content/uploads/sites/2/2016/04/Call-to-Action-Unicef-UK-Baby-Friendly-Initiative.pdf

Unicef UK (2016b) Transition guidance: Moving from the current to the new Baby Friendly Initiative standards, https://www.unicef.org.uk/wp-content/uploads/sites/2/2016/08/transition_guidance.pdf

Unicef UK (2016c) Achieving sustainability: Standards and guidance, https://www.unicef.org.uk/babyfriendly/baby-friendly-resources/guidance-for-health-professionals/implementing-the-baby-friendly-standards/achieving-sustainability-standards-guidance/

Unicef UK (2017a) 'Awards table: Baby Friendly services near me', https://www.unicef.org.uk/babyfriendly/what-is-baby-friendly/breastfeeding-in-the-uk/baby-friendly-services-near-me/

Unicef UK (2017b) Removing the barriers to breastfeeding: A call to action, https://www.unicef.org.uk/babyfriendly/wp-content/uploads/sites/2/2017/07/Barriers-to-Breastfeeding-Briefing-The-Baby-Friendly-Initiative.pdf

Victora, C. G., Bahl, R., Barros, A.J.D., França, G.V.A., Horton, S., Krasevec, J., Murch, S, Sankar, M. J., Walker, N., Rollins, N. C., on behalf of The Lancet Breastfeeding Series Group (2016) 'Breastfeeding in the 21st century: epidemiology, mechanisms, and lifelong effect', *Lancet*, 387(10017): 403–504

WHO/Unicef (1989) *Protecting, promoting and supporting breastfeeding: The special role of maternity services*, Geneva: WHO and Unicef.

WHO/Unicef (1992) 'National implementation of the Baby-friendly Hospital Initiative', Geneva: WHO/Unicef, http://apps.who.int/iris/bitstream/10665/255197/1/9789241512381-eng.pdf?ua=1

WHO (2017) 'Protecting, promoting and supporting breastfeeding in facilities providing maternity and newborn services', Geneva: WHO: http://www.who.int/nutrition/publications/guidelines/breastfeeding-facilities-maternity-newborn/en/

Wright, S. (1998) 'Politicisation of "culture"', *Anthropology in Action*, 5: 3–10.

PART I

Breastfeeding and emotions

ONE

Managing the dynamics of shame in breastfeeding support

Dawn Leeming

Introduction

Our society has such a conflicted approach to breastfeeding that not only can women feel shamed for breastfeeding, they can also be shamed for not breastfeeding (Thomson et al, 2015). On the one hand, concerns about public feeding can invoke embarrassment or sexual shame about exposure for women, as well as feelings of disgust about visible lactation and hence shame about *being* disgusting (Dowling et al, 2012). On the other hand, women can feel shame when they decide not to breastfeed or find it difficult to establish breastfeeding (see the meta-synthesis by Burns et al, 2010).

In this chapter I examine research on women's experiences of breastfeeding which explores how shame might arise where they face challenges with this. I then consider what might be learned about breastfeeding support from a body of literature that has previously been overlooked in relation to infant feeding: the literature on shame and shame resilience. Exploring the differences between shame (feeling lesser in some way and unworthy of acceptance) and guilt (the sense that one has done something wrong), I explain why shame is more likely than guilt to lead to interpersonal problems, including difficulties in receiving support. The key argument in this chapter is that it is important to broaden the discussion of the emotional impact of not meeting breastfeeding expectations beyond the consideration of guilt (Taylor and Wallace, 2012). In doing so, those supporting and promoting breastfeeding can become attuned to the trickier interpersonal dynamics of shame and the sociocultural contexts which produce it.

The hidden nature of shame

It is only recently that breastfeeding researchers have turned their attention to shame (for example, Taylor and Wallace, 2012; Thomson et al, 2015). This may be because we do not often talk about shame in Western societies. We have become ashamed of our shame (Scheff, 2003), so that research on issues related to shame (for example, stigma, fear of rejection, fear of negative evaluation, lack of self-worth) does not often use the 'S word' (Scheff and Mateo, 2016). The literature on shame management and self-presentation (for example, Nathanson, 1997; Schlenker, 2012) also suggests that we often work hard to *avoid* shame. We may do this in a number of ways, such as constructing and presenting a desired identity, seeking affirmation, and saving face by concealment or strategic use of excuses, justifications, apologies and blame. However, the possibility of shame often remains unspoken while we do this, and we may manage shame by denying we feel any, or we simply may not have the language to discuss it (Brown, 2006). This relative invisibility of the feeling means that we have to listen carefully to what women say and do in relation to breastfeeding if we are going to be sensitive to signs of shame.

The relevance of shame to breastfeeding

The relevance of shame to some women's experiences of breastfeeding is suggested by themes of self-blame, inadequacy and failure identified in the accounts of women who have experienced breastfeeding difficulty during the early weeks and later (Mozingo et al, 2000; Guyer et al, 2012; Williamson et al, 2012; Thomson et al, 2015; see also Smyth, Chapter Two in this volume). The following quotes are from a UK study in which we interviewed new mothers intending to breastfeed, and asked them to keep audio-diaries of their feeding experiences during the first few weeks:

> 'I just cried and cried and cried 'cos it was just such a big disappointment I felt like I had failed really, almost as a woman really, you feel like this is a natural thing, why can I not do this?'
>
> 'It [topping up with a bottle of formula milk] also made me feel very, um, just like a really crap mother, to be honest ... I just felt that I couldn't um, produce what she was needing ... It just made me feel very inadequate.' (Williamson et al, 2012: 440).

Several of the mothers in the study struggled to establish breastfeeding. Some found it difficult to establish a good attachment of the baby to the breast, or experienced pain, or found that their baby was disinterested in breastfeeding or unsettled. Breastfeeding difficulties are not uncommon in the UK in the early weeks (McAndrew et al, 2012), and it is therefore worth considering why these women might understand such difficulties as a personal shortcoming – a sign that they had failed and were inadequate as mothers.

Mothering has been found to be one of the most common shame triggers for women (Brown, 2006). Taylor and Wallace (2012) draw on Wolf's idea of total motherhood (Wolf, 2007) to suggest that women may be vulnerable to shame around mothering where they are encouraged to focus entirely on optimising children's wellbeing with no space for their own needs, so that perfection is demanded. Women may then feel an overwhelming *duty* to breastfeed rather than consider that they have a health-related *reason* to do so (Woollard, 2016). A sense of failure then becomes difficult to avoid if breastfeeding goals and expectations are not fully met and, regardless of the contextual constraints on a woman's experience of breastfeeding (for example, lack of advice about latching problems, or family disapproval of breastfeeding), not meeting ideals is likely to become internalised as personal shame and guilt.

Several studies have suggested that breastfeeding is an area of motherhood where there may be a particular gap between expectations and reality due to limited prenatal discussion of potential difficulties (Larsen et al, 2008; Burns et al, 2010; Hoddinott et al, 2012). Women may be even more likely to see their postnatal feeding difficulties as a personal flaw without sufficient prior information to make sense of the problem (Williamson et al, 2012). The second quotation cited earlier suggests that this gap between expectations and reality can become particularly problematic if women's expectations are based on a view of the 'good mother' as an embodied phenomenon who does not just breastfeed but lactates plentifully and sustains her child with ease. From the perspective of this participant, she *was* her inadequately lactating body: "*I* couldn't produce what she was needing," not, "*my body* didn't produce" (Williamson et al, 2012). Although some women talked about the breastfeeding body in a more distanced and even mechanical way, several women who were struggling to establish breastfeeding talked more holistically about connections between their bodies and selves in ways which were very self-denigrating. They interpreted experiencing pain, or difficulties latching the baby to the breast, or perceiving that their milk supply was inadequate, as meaning that they were not normal because breastfeeding was supposed to be a 'natural' part of being a mother (Williamson et al, 2012). The first quote cited earlier also suggests that the speaker interpreted her difficulties with lactation as an assault on her femininity, as well as on her identity as a mother: "I felt like I had failed really, almost as a woman." Taylor and Wallace (2012) note that promoting breastfeeding by linking breastfeeding and femininity can contribute to shame by positioning non-breastfeeding women as less feminine. As Smyth explains in the next chapter, perceived failure can then be experienced as if it calls the status of the self into question.

Shame versus guilt

Distress about not breastfeeding has sometimes been discussed as guilt, so it is worth exploring the differences between shame and guilt to establish clarity. Both guilt and shame are probably best understood as fuzzy categories of experience which can overlap and be experienced together (Blum, 2008) as part of a family of related feelings that also includes embarrassment and humiliation (Scheff, 2003). Although there is some degree of overlap, research suggests that there are some important differences between the experiences that people label primarily as shame, and those experiences that they label primarily as guilt. However, theorists have argued in the literature about the best way to capture these differences.

The most common distinction made between shame and guilt (Tangney and Dearing, 2002; Tracy and Robins, 2004) is between making a negative judgement of our whole self (shame) versus a negative judgement that our behaviour has not met moral standards (guilt). Using this distinction, then, shame might arise if a woman sees herself as a bad mother or a failure as a woman, whereas guilt would arise if she made a negative judgement about a particular way she had behaved – for example, she may consider that she has done something wrong by not breastfeeding. From this perspective, shame is the more problematic emotion because of the resulting sense of a worthless, disabled self. Van Vliet (2008) talks about shame as an assault on the self or 'a shattering of who I am'.

Other theorists (Scheff, 2003; Elison, 2005) emphasise the interpersonal features of shame and view awareness of devaluation or a threat to social bonds as crucial for shame, rather than negative *self*-evaluation. They view guilt, on the other hand, as simply awareness of wrongdoing, and this may or may not be associated with devaluation and concurrent shame. From this perspective, when we are ashamed we have a sense of a bad or flawed self, and of this self being exposed before others. We see ourselves through the eyes of others, for example, as if there is a socially shared understanding that we are a bad mother. This perspective suggests that the difficulty with shame arises from a sense that we have lost the acceptance of others and our sense of connection with others.

A particularly useful model of shame and guilt has been developed by Gilbert (Gilbert et al, 1994; Gilbert, 2003), who drew on the work of Lewis (1971) to integrate some of these varied ideas about shame and guilt. He suggests that there are different interpersonal processes in guilt and shame, and argues that the two experiences differ in the way power inequalities are felt. When we feel guilt, we focus on others as victims of our actions and see the other (for example the baby) as hurt and needy, and ourselves as the one with the power to hurt. Because we see ourselves as responsible for the situation, we focus not just on our specific actions or inactions and what was wrong with these, but on how to put things right. However, when we feel shame, we feel powerless and incapable of remedying the situation. It is the other (for example, someone observing our mothering) that seems stronger and more able as we shrink before their scorn. We have a painful sense of ourselves through others' eyes as 'bad', or as being an object of ridicule or inadequacy. Gilbert notes that this 'other' need not necessarily be an actual other. We may feel ashamed in front of an internalised sense of a general other – a sense of being exposed as inadequate with an unwanted identity. We therefore experience ourselves as inferior. If the experience of shame is intense, we might feel physically uncomfortable (hot, sick, blushing) and helpless, paralysed and unable to think clearly beyond wanting to shrink, flee or hide our bad self from possible exposure and judgement. Transient feelings of shame may not necessarily be this strong, and we are sometimes very good at resisting or deflecting shame because it is so painful. However, Gilbert's model highlights the way that any sense of a shamefully exposed or flawed self is difficult to manage because it is not just a feeling, but a sense of a devalued position in the world from which it is difficult to escape or remedy the situation.

How shame may lead to tricky interpersonal processes

While shame is clearly an issue for some breastfeeding women, there is danger in overstating the possibility of shame for all women. Not every mother who experiences breastfeeding challenges internalises these struggles, and not every mother is troubled by the possibility of negative judgement by others. Mothers are not passive recipients of cultural representations around infant feeding. They carefully weigh up the information that is given to them and the ideas of those people who are close to them. Sometimes they actively renegotiate the definitions of 'good mothering' in order to resist the ideals that suggest they might be failing in some way (Marshall et al, 2007). This identity work could be considered a form of shame management or avoidance, but it can be burdensome emotion-work and can invoke tricky interpersonal processes which are likely to work against gaining support with breastfeeding.

Several responses to shame can amplify people's feelings and further damage relationships with others (Nathanson, 1997; Elison et al, 2006). Three of these responses seem particularly relevant to the current discussion. First, women might castigate themselves further for their struggles with breastfeeding and build a spiral of shame (Kaufman, 1992). In a spiral of shame people become more and more focused on their inadequacies, and replay shaming scenes. This can lead them to become less and less able to connect meaningfully with the external world, and can result in the second response of withdrawal, hiding or isolation (Nathanson, 1997). Hiding avoids the further exposure of people's perceived inadequacies. People who find shame very difficult to tolerate might withdraw from others at the first thought of failure or judgement in order to avoid the experience of shame. It is not difficult to imagine that someone who fears that her difficulties with breastfeeding might mean she is not a good mother, and who is acutely embarrassed at exposing what she sees as 'malfunctioning' nipples, might prefer to withdraw from the support offered. She might attempt to manage alone using strategies such as topping up with infant formula or relying on expressed breast milk given through a bottle. This may seem preferable to seeking help with feeding at the breast. Thomson, Ebisch-Burton and Flacking (2015) noted that some women in their study were reluctant to seek help with breastfeeding if they thought others might perceive them as being unable to cope, and withdrew from others following perceived criticism.

An alternative response to withdrawal or self-attack when we sense the possibility of shame is to attack others (Nathanson, 1997). Responding to perceived devaluation by blaming or criticising others, or by becoming overtly angry and hostile, is sometimes known as 'humiliated fury' (Lewis, 1971). Shame is more likely to lead to anger, hostility and distance from others when it is not acknowledged (Scheff and Retzinger, 1991; Scheff, 1995). Instead of openly and respectfully discussing another person's disapproval or challenge, the person who perceives they are being criticised or treated disrespectfully defends their self against feelings of shame by also engaging in subtly disrespectful behaviour (for example, disengagement or belittling) which in turn shames the other person and can lead to perpetuating cycles of mutual unacknowledged shame, anger and conflict.

Scheff and Retzinger provide detailed analyses of unacknowledged shaming interactions that may take place in psychotherapy (for example, Retzinger, 1998), but Lazare (1987) is one of the few to apply these ideas about unacknowledged shame to healthcare consultations. He notes that there is the potential for shame in healthcare settings where patients may feel exposed, vulnerable and scrutinised, and they may believe that their healthcare problem is a defect or shortcoming. These ideas have a clear resonance for our understanding of breastfeeding and women seeking help with breastfeeding (Thomson et al, 2015). Lazare argues that some of the difficult behaviours that are encountered in healthcare settings can be understood as a response to shame and part of unspoken shame cycles. He cites examples of behaviour from service users that might seem difficult or disrespectful, such as being late, missing appointments, withholding information and even complaining to others about the healthcare professional. Healthcare professionals and breastfeeding supporters are themselves not immune to involvement in shame cycles. A client who withdraws or does not engage with healthcare advice, or is even critical and attacking, can leave the healthcare professional feeling a sense of failure or inadequacy. There is the possibility that health professionals then defend themselves against this by blaming the client. Lazare argues that it is important for healthcare professionals to be aware of shame dynamics and to avoid a disrespectful response to difficult clients. This analysis has been extended by Gray (2009) and Gibson (2015) with regard to substance abuse counselling and child protection, respectively. They suggest that an overly directive and/or coercive stance may also inadvertently shame clients. This can dehumanise the client and invalidate his or her viewpoint (Gray, 2009), and may result in withdrawal or resistance to services (Gibson, 2015).

Guilt has been seen as the unwanted emotional side effect of breastfeeding promotion (Williams et al, 2012), but there are reasons to believe, from the analyses of Lazare and others, that shame might be more problematic than guilt for some women who experience difficulties with breastfeeding and internalise them as a mark of failure or invalidation of their mothering. Shame can derail relationships with supporters of breastfeeding, leading to withdrawal or resistance. Shame may also be a greater challenge to wellbeing than guilt, as chronic and pervasive shame may seriously challenge a woman's mental health (Tangney and Dearing, 2002). Clearly shame is not necessarily an issue for all women seeking support with breastfeeding, and many women focus on breastfeeding as a source of satisfaction, achievement and meaningful connection with their baby (Burns et al, 2010; see also Smyth, Chapter Two in this volume). However, where the possibility of shame arises, it is important to consider how this can be resisted, and how women might be supported in developing resilience in the face of shame.

Helping new mothers resist and avoid feeling shamed by breastfeeding difficulties

Realistic breastfeeding promotion and education

Resisting shame is highly relevant to Hausman's (2012) and Trickey's (2016) arguments that the promotion of breastfeeding should shift away from emphasising the individual mother's responsibility to make better choices (mothers already know that breast is best for health) and place greater emphasis on challenging the constraints on women's *right* to breastfeed. The first emphasis shames mothers; the second does not and recognises the social and material realities that may work against breastfeeding. The environmental constraints on breastfeeding are indicated by the marked differences in breastfeeding rates between different geographical areas, according to relative levels of deprivation (Brown et al, 2010). Several chapters in this volume also note the cultural taboos which limit breastfeeding (see Chapters Two, Three and Four). Hausman (2007) points out that most leisure and work spaces are set up with male norms, which assume that adults will not have a baby attached to their body. Following such thinking, the recent Unicef UK campaign addresses anti-breastfeeding cultures and social structures, rather than 'laying the blame for a major public health issue on individual women' (Unicef UK, 2016a). Such an ecological approach, which theorises infant feeding as a sociocultural phenomenon embedded within broader systems, may identify and address the constraints on breastfeeding, and may also reduce the shame and guilt where women struggle with breastfeeding because of these constraints (Trickey, 2016).

Cultural taboos contribute to the relative invisibility of breastfeeding and the almost total invisibility of human milk. Many first-time mothers have not watched another mother breastfeed, never mind observed a mother struggling to adjust the positioning of her nipple and her baby while milk spurts in all directions, which leads to idealised expectations. As Taylor and Wallace have argued, a greater variety of embodied breastfeeding experiences needs to be acknowledged – 'be they good, bad or even ugly' (2012: 201). This would ensure that the promotion of idyllic and idealised images of breastfeeding does not shame women who find that their experience does not fit with these images, particularly in the early days. Hoddinott et al (2012), among others, have argued for a more woman-centred and realistic approach to promoting breastfeeding, which acknowledges the difficulties and accepts that sometimes goals may need to be modified. This seems a useful approach, though any normalising of breastfeeding difficulties needs careful handling in case this reinforces the idea that breastfeeding is *inherently* difficult and discourages women from breastfeeding. Women are aware that breastfeeding is considered to be 'natural', but we also need to promote the message that this does not necessarily mean that the act of breastfeeding is immediately obvious to mothers and babies. Otherwise women will continue to make sense of breastfeeding difficulties as if these are their personal shortcomings. Trickey and Newburn (2014) have suggested stronger promotion of the idea of an adjustment period in breastfeeding, which seems to be a useful approach.

Supporting mothers in becoming resilient against shame

In an ideal world, women would begin breastfeeding after they had observed other women breastfeed. They would be aware of the breastfeeding challenges they may face in the early days and would have immediate support to deal with these. Also, they would live in a cultural setting where they had space and time to concentrate on feeding their babies. In this ideal world, they would not be trying to learn a new and mysterious skill while hiding under a blanket, and we might expect lactation challenges to be fewer and more easily overcome. While Western social conditions often do not meet these standards, some degree of difficulty with breastfeeding can be expected for some women. Therefore, it is important to consider how women and their babies may be supported in learning to breastfeed. However, this is unlikely to be sufficient on its own without also helping women to manage their emotional responses to breastfeeding challenges. If we can also support women emotionally, we may reduce shame-related phenomena such as withdrawal, helplessness, hopelessness and hostile interactions that prevent mothers from getting the help and support they need.

A useful resource for developing emotional support is the recent qualitative research on shame resilience and repair of shame (Brown, 2006; Van Vliet, 2008; Leeming and Boyle, 2013; Dayal et al, 2015). This research is not specifically focused on breastfeeding, but it emphasises the importance of interpersonal processes in managing shame and is useful for thinking about how we may support breastfeeding women. Shame involves a sense of being disconnected from others, and this research suggests that a key process in repairing shame is restoring a person's sense of meaningful connection with others (Brown, 2006; Van Vliet, 2008; Dayal et al, 2015). Closely related to this is a person's sense of being accepted by others – a sense of validation, such that you and your experiences *matter* to someone (Leeming and Boyle, 2013). We can tolerate and repair shame more easily if we have a sense that others value us (Leeming and Boyle, 2013), that they have an empathic understanding of our perspective (Brown, 2006), and that they are likely to provide a safe space for us to disclose what we see as shameful aspects of ourselves (Dayal et al, 2015).

It's interesting that these issues – connection, acceptance, validation – have already been identified as important in breastfeeding support. A meta-synthesis of women's experiences of breastfeeding support demonstrated that 'authentic presence' – a meaningful relationship with those supporting their breastfeeding – was highly valued by mothers (Schmied et al, 2011). Although mothers preferred supporters spending time with them, even brief contact could demonstrate that supporters took an interest and considered the mothers' experiences to be important. This 'authentic presence' also included providing reassurance and positive affirmation of the women's mothering, and seems similar to helpful responses to shame identified in previous research, which enabled the shamed individual to reposition themselves positively in relation to others (Leeming and Boyle, 2013). Van Vliet (2008) argues that this repositioning is important in 'rebuilding the self'. We do not know how many of the women contributing data to the meta-synthesis *had* struggled with breastfeeding difficulties and feelings of inadequacy in relation to this. However, it seems reasonable to assume, based on research discussed earlier, that some of them would have felt this and that 'authentic presence' might have been valued by some *because* it helped them to resist potential feelings of shame. Connection and validation are also likely to be important factors for women in deciding whether contact with other breastfeeding women may be helpful, or potentially exposing. It is easy to imagine how you might feel if you were on the margins of a peer support group where everyone else appeared to be getting the hang of breastfeeding except you, and how this could be experienced as quite shaming rather than empowering and supportive. Positive and affirming relationships within the group are likely to be crucial for avoiding this.

One of the strongest messages coming from the shame resilience research is that secrecy and silence rarely help to repair shame. If someone seems embarrassed, guilty or ashamed, we tend to avoid referring to the source of these feelings, but this can be taken as legitimising the sense of shame (Gibson, 2015). Articulating or 'speaking' shame is often essential for someone to tolerate what she sees as a less than perfect or less than hoped for aspect of herself (Brown, 2006). This enables her to see that she is still valued by others despite the exposure of what she perceives as inadequacies, and her shame about this. Without speaking about what we see as shameful aspects of ourselves (whether these are our capabilities, our bodies or our circumstances) it becomes difficult to see these aspects as quite possibly normal. The small body of research on repairing shame strongly suggests that speaking about things that shame us can help us to examine our assumptions and conclusions and hear alternative views which contextualise the issue differently. A re-contextualisation might involve examining or critiquing the cultural norms and assumptions which shame us, and the wider political context which restricts individual choice. For example, what is seen as failure to meet the 'good mother' ideal of breastfeeding with ease could be re-contextualised in a less shaming manner. It could include an understanding of the anatomy and physiology of breastfeeding (the difficulties of fitting a particular mouth to a particular breast), and the impact of work, leisure and other public environments that take male embodiment as the norm (Hausman, 2007) and constrain good lactation management.

If women feel comfortable enough to articulate with infant feeding supporters any feelings they may have of shame, failure or self-denigration, then this places the feelings out in the world where they can be accepted as feelings that matter, and gently examined and challenged. This seems a more productive way forward than women ruminating privately, being drawn into a spiral of shame and withdrawing from sources of support or becoming hostile and defensive. The recent Baby Friendly Initiative guidance on having meaningful conversations with mothers seems useful in this respect (Unicef, 2016b). It suggests that breastfeeding supporters should ask open questions about feelings, show empathy, use active listening and avoid overt direction and judgement. This guidance also fits with a more person-centred approach to breastfeeding support (Dykes, 2006), which emphasises empowerment and valuing women, and minimising the potential for women to feel scrutinised and evaluated. Infant feeding supporters also need to remain sensitive to signs of shame or shame avoidance in their conversations with mothers. Gibson (2015) notes that shame is usually referred to indirectly and clients are likely to find it difficult to articulate their shame. Therefore, he argues, supporters need to note signs such as defensiveness, withdrawal, avoidance of eye contact or other hiding behaviours, hesitation, self-censorship, negative self-evaluation and inauthentic smiling. Good 'shame antennae' are needed when supporting mothers from marginalised groups who may already feel they are stigmatised and assume their mothering is under more critical professional surveillance if they are, for example, younger or older mothers, mothers from groups with minority parenting norms, mothers experiencing social deprivation, or mothers with mental health difficulties.

Conclusion

Paying attention to shame dynamics is important when we are supporting women who are breastfeeding their babies, because this is an aspect of mothering that is heavily moralised and scrutinised through an ideological lens that values certain feminine behaviours and shames others. Some of the current approaches to breastfeeding support seem attuned to these sensitivities but don't fully articulate the importance of shame resilience. However, in bringing issues of shame to the fore, there is a risk that talking about shame may locate the 'problem' within breastfeeding women. We may inadvertently reinforce the idea that breastfeeding is somehow shameful by focusing on women's emotional responses instead of focusing on the competing and unrealistic expectations that are placed on mothers, and the social and cultural constraints that are placed on breastfeeding. Taylor and Wallace point out that 'the fear of inducing maternal guilt [in relation to breastfeeding] has become a trope that provides a politically effective way of appearing to care about mothers without actually having to do anything concrete to assist them' (Taylor and Wallace, 2012: 196). We should be careful that the same does not happen with shame.

I argue here that an interpersonal approach to shame is useful for considering the dynamics between mothers and breastfeeding advocates and support workers. However, it is vital that we also conceptualise shame within a broader understanding of the cultural discourses (and absences of discourse) that shame breastfeeding women. We must promote an understanding of the breastfeeding challenges that shame some women that focuses clearly on the male-centred norms, institutions and public spaces that interfere with lactation. Shame can feel the most personal and private of experiences, but to address it we need to turn to the wider social context.

References

Blum, A. (2008) 'Shame and guilt, misconceptions and controversies: a critical review of the literature', *Traumatology*, 14(3): 91–102.

Brown, B. (2006) 'Shame resilience theory: a grounded theory study on women and shame', *Families in Society: The Journal of Contemporary Social Services*, 87(1): 43–52.

Brown, A. E., Raynor, P., Benton, D. and Lee, M. D. (2010) 'Indices of multiple deprivation predict breastfeeding duration in England and Wales', *European Journal of Public Health*, 20(2): 231–5.

Burns, E., Schmied, V., Sheehan, A. and Fenwick, J. (2010) 'A meta-ethnographic synthesis of women's experience of breastfeeding', *Maternal and Child Nutrition*, 6(3): 201–19.

Dayal, H., Weaver, K. and Domene, J. F. (2015) 'From shame to shame resilience: narratives of counsellor trainees with eating issues', *Qualitative Health Research*, 25(2): 153–67.

Dowling, S., Naidoo, J. and Pontin, D. (2012) 'Breastfeeding in public: women's bodies, women's milk', in P. Hall Smith, B. L. Hausman, and M. Labbok (eds) *Beyond health, beyond choice: Breastfeeding constraints and realities*, Chapel Hill: Rutgers Press, pp 249–58.

Dykes, F. (2006) 'The education of health practitioners supporting breastfeeding women: time for critical reflection', *Maternal and Child Nutrition*, 2(4): 204–16.

Elison, J. (2005) 'Shame and guilt: a hundred years of apples and oranges', *New Ideas in Psychology*, 23(5): 5–32.

Elison, J., Pulos, S. and Lennon, R. (2006) 'Shame-focused coping: an empirical study of the compass of shame', *Social Behavior and Personality*, 34(2): 161–8.

Gibson, M. (2015) 'Shame and guilt in child protection social work: new interpretations and opportunities for practice', *Child and Family Social Work*, 20(3): 333–43.

Gilbert, P. (2003) 'Evolution, social roles, and the differences in shame and guilt', *Social Research*, 70(4): 1205–30.

Gilbert, P., Pehl, J. and Allan, S. (1994) 'The phenomenology of shame and guilt: an empirical investigation', *British Journal of Medical Psychology*, 67(1): 23–36.

Gray, R. (2009) 'The dynamics of shame: implications for counsellors working in alcohol and other drug settings', *Psychotherapy in Australia*, 16(1): 30–36.

Guyer, J., Millward, L. J. and Berger, I. (2012) 'Mothers' breastfeeding experiences and implications for professionals', *British Journal of Midwifery*, 20(10): 724–32.

Hausman, B. (2007) 'Things (not) to do with breasts in public: maternal embodiment and the biocultural politics of infant feeding', *New Literary History*, 38(3): 479–504.

Hausman, B. (2012) 'Feminism and breastfeeding: rhetoric, ideology, and the maternal realities of women's lives', in P. Hall Smith, B. L. Hausman and M. Labbok (eds) *Beyond health, beyond choice: Breastfeeding constraints and realities*, Chapel Hill: Rutgers Press, pp 15–24.

Hoddinott, P., Craig, L.C.A., Britten, J. and McInnes, R. M. (2012) 'A serial qualitative interview study of infant feeding experiences: idealism meets realism', *BMJ Open*, 2(2): e000504.

Kaufman, G. (1992) *Shame: The power of caring*, New York: Schenkman Books.

Larsen, J. S., Hall, E.O.C. and Aagaard, H. (2008) 'Shattered expectations: when mothers' confidence in breastfeeding is undermined – a metasynthesis', *Scandinavian Journal of Caring Science*, 22(4): 653–61.

Lazare, A. (1987) 'Shame and humiliation in the medical encounter', *Archives of Internal Medicine*, 147(9): 1653–8.

Leeming, D. and Boyle, M. (2013) 'Managing shame: an interpersonal perspective', *British Journal of Social Psychology*, 52(1): 140–60.

Lewis, H. B. (1971) *Shame and guilt in neurosis*, New York: International Universities Press.

Marshall, J. L., Godfrey, M. and Renfrew, M. J. (2007) 'Being a "good mother": managing breastfeeding and merging identities', *Social Science and Medicine*, 65(10): 2147–59.

McAndrew, F., Thompson, J., Fellows, L., Large, A., Speed, M. and Renfrew, M. (2012) 'Infant Feeding Survey 2010', London: Health and Social Care Information Centre, http://content.digital.nhs.uk/catalogue/PUB08694/Infant-Feeding-Survey-2010-Consolidated-Report.pdf

Mozingo, J. N., Davis, M. W., Droppleman, P. G. and Merideth, A. (2000) '"It wasn't working": women's experiences with short-term breastfeeding', *MCN: The American Journal of Maternal Child Nursing*, 25(3): 120–26.

Nathanson, D. L. (1997) 'Affect theory and the compass of shame', in M. R. Lansky and A. P. Morrison (eds) *The widening scope of shame*, Hillsdale, NJ: Analytic Press, pp 339–54.

Retzinger, S. (1998) 'Shame in the therapeutic relationship', in P. Gilbert and B. Andrews (eds) *Shame: Interpersonal behavior, psychopathology, and culture*, New York: Oxford University Press, pp 206–22.

Scheff, T. J. (1995) 'Conflict in family systems: the role of shame', in J. P. Tangney and K. W. Fischer (eds) *Self-conscious emotions: The psychology of shame, guilt, embarrassment and pride*, New York: Guilford Press, pp 393–412.

Scheff, T. J. (2003) 'Shame in self and society', *Symbolic Interaction*, 26(2): 239–62.

Scheff, T. J. and Mateo, S. (2016) 'The S-word is taboo: shame is invisible in modern societies', *Journal of General Practice*, 4(1): 217.

Scheff, T. J. and Retzinger, S. (1991) *Emotions and violence: Shame and rage in destructive conflict*, New York: Lexington.

Schlenker, B. (2012) 'Self-presentation', in M. R. Leary and J. P. Tangney (eds) *Handbook of self and identity* (2nd edn), New York: Guildford Press, pp 542–70.

Schmied, V., Beake, S., Sheehan, A., McCourt, C. and Dykes, F. (2011), 'Women's perceptions and experiences of breastfeeding support: a metasynthesis', *BIRTH*, 38(1): 49–60.

Tangney, J. P. and Dearing, R. L. (2002) *Shame and guilt*, New York: Guilford Press.

Taylor, E. N. and Wallace, L. E. (2012) 'Feminist breastfeeding advocacy and the problem of guilt', in P. Hall Smith, B. L. Hausman, and M. Labbok (eds) *Beyond health, beyond choice: Breastfeeding constraints and realities*, Chapel Hill: Rutgers Press, pp 193–202.

Thomson, G., Ebisch-Burton, K. and Flacking, R. (2015), 'Shame if you do – shame if you don't: women's experiences of infant feeding', *Maternal and Child Nutrition*, 11(1): 33–46.

Tracy, J. L. and Robins, R. W. (2004) 'Putting the self into self-conscious emotions: a theoretical model', *Psychological Inquiry*, 15(2): 103–25.

Trickey, H. (2016) 'Changing the conversation: ecological thinking', *Perspective*, 33(Dec).

Trickey, H. and Newburn, M. (2014) 'Goals, dilemmas and assumptions in infant feeding education and support: applying theory of constraints thinking tools to develop new priorities for action', *Maternal and Child Nutrition*, 10(1): 72–91.

Unicef UK (2016a) 'Protecting health and saving lives: A call to action', https://www.unicef.org.uk/babyfriendly/baby-friendly-resources/advocacy/join-our-change-the-conversation-campaign

Unicef UK (2016b) 'Having meaningful conversations with mothers: A guide to using the Baby Friendly signature sheets', https://www.unicef.org.uk/babyfriendly/wp-content/uploads/sites/2/2016/10/meaningful_conversations.pdf

Van Vliet, K. J. (2008) 'Shame and resilience in adulthood: a grounded theory study', *Journal of Counselling Psychology*, 55(2): 233–45.

Williams, K., Donaghue, N. and Kurz, T. (2012) '"Giving guilt the flick?": an investigation of mothers' talk about guilt in relation to infant feeding', *Psychology of Women Quarterly*, 37(1): 97–112.

Williamson, I., Leeming, D., Lyttle, S. and Johnson, S. (2012) '"It should be the most natural thing in the world": exploring first-time mothers' breastfeeding difficulties in the UK using audio-diaries and interviews', *Maternal and Child Nutrition*, 8(4): 434–47.

Wolf, J.B. (2007) 'Is breast really best? Risk and total motherhood in the National Breastfeeding Awareness Campaign', *Journal of Health Politics, Policy and Law*, 32(4): 595–636.

Woollard, F. (2016) 'Changing the conversation: reasons not duties', *Perspective*, 33(Dec).

TWO

Breastfeeding's emotional intensity: pride, shame and status

Lisa Smyth

Introduction

> It's time that we abandon simple solutions and simple slogans, and grapple with the nuance. (Hinde, 2017)

Breastfeeding has become a major global public health priority, with concerted efforts well underway to raise rates across the world (WHO and Unicef, 1989; WHO, 2003). However, only 37% of infants on average are exclusively breastfed at six months in low- and middle-income countries, where the protective effects of breastfeeding for infant and child health are well known. Over 80% of infants are initially breastfed at birth in high-income countries but by the end of the first year, this has dropped to an average of 20%. The UK has one of the lowest rates in the world, with less than 1% of infants breastfed at 12 months in 2010 (McAndrew et al, 2012), in contrast to 27% in the US and 35% in Norway (Victora et al, 2016). The relationship between breastfeeding and global economic inequality is clear from the recent comparative work carried out by Victora et al, which demonstrates that 'for each doubling in the gross domestic product per head, breastfeeding prevalence at 12 months decreased by ten percentage points' (Victora et al, 2016: 477).

Local inequalities also shape patterns of breastfeeding. The relationship between rates of sustained breastfeeding and patterns of inequality are well known within the UK (McAndrew et al, 2012). Those most likely to breastfeed are mothers from all minority ethnic backgrounds, and women aged 30 or over in managerial or professional occupations with educational qualifications beyond second level (McAndrew et al, 2012). Regional dynamics are also significant: Northern Ireland has the lowest rates of breastfeeding of the four UK countries, and consequently the world.

Public health researchers have examined the relationship between breastfeeding attitudes and social inequalities (Miracle and Fredland, 2007; Strong, 2013), the physical challenges to breastfeeding (Kelleher, 2006; Ryan et al, 2013), and the effects of medicalisation (Thompson et al, 2011). Emotional support from family and friends (Wambach and Cohen, 2009), and practical support from health professionals, male partners and employers is important for developing effective interventions to improve breastfeeding rates (Chuang et al, 2010; Dykes and Flacking, 2010; Van Wagenen et al, 2015). These studies show that infant feeding practices are shaped by interpersonal and more general, public social relations (Dykes and Flacking, 2010; Callaghan and Lazard, 2011; Dowling et al, 2012). What is less well understood is how underlying social processes of status inequality, anxiety and shame shape infant feeding orientation. This chapter examines this connection by looking at the ways in which status anxiety experienced through shame makes infant feeding an emotionally intense feature of early mothering (Taylor and Wallace, 2012b).

Status anxiety

Our health and wellbeing are shaped by our socioeconomic class, and by our social status. While economic class is an important form of inequality, it works together with status, which is a less tangible but powerful form of social differentiation (Turner, 1988). The social theorist Max Weber defined status as 'a specific, positive or negative, social estimation of honour' (Weber, 1978: 932). This 'honour', or esteem (Brennan and Pettit, 2004), is attached to identities which are ascribed to us because of our gender, ethnicity or age, as well as the identities that we achieve, for example, through education, sport or music. Status takes objective and subjective forms and involves public recognition of esteem, for instance, through number of 'likes' on Facebook and our perceptions of how well others regard us as we perform our social roles, such as mother or friend.

The effort not to lose esteem by 'falling behind' or 'losing face' is a crucial motivation that shapes what we do and how we feel about ourselves (Goffman, 1971 [1956]; Frank, 2007). Being able to meet the ordinary standards of our social context is an everyday priority, if we are to avoid feeling bad about ourselves (Frank, 2007). Having a sense of what is expected of someone 'like me', and a record of behaving accordingly (Stewart, 1994) is crucial in securing or maintaining status.

These felt estimations of esteem tend to focus on our style of living relative to the people around us, rather than how much income or wealth we might have. For example, we might seek esteem from the location and decor of our home, from our style of dress, use of language, musical taste or family size (Chan and Goldthorpe, 2007). A young woman's expectation of how she would be esteemed for the way she dresses when she goes clubbing is different from how she might expect to be esteemed for how she dresses while caring for her young children.

We are all caught up in these endless processes of judging each other and ourselves in the light of wider expectations about people 'like us' – recognising, withdrawing, and claiming status in the form of esteem as we go about our daily lives (McBride, 2013). To do this we rely on status symbols, such as dress or language, and by showing how well we meet social expectations through the competence we display as we act, for example, as a new mother (Sunstein, 1996). However, displays of status symbols or competent role performances cannot guarantee status, and the uncertainty generates a pressure on our everyday behaviour (Goffman, 1951). Anxiety about our status becomes severe when a social role combines incompatible expectations. The intense pressure experienced by mothers in paid employment goes beyond the practical strain of juggling paid and unpaid work in societies where the norm of the male breadwinner is strong. Mothers in employment routinely meet expectations that the good worker is totally devoted to employment, while the good mother is devoted to raising her children; these tensions can have significant effects on job/ career prospects, wellbeing and family life (Blair-Loy, 2003; Ridgeway and Correll, 2004; Lewis et al, 2008; Benard and Correll, 2010).

While status and economic class may be closely intertwined, they work differently and may have distinct effects (Turner, 1988). Rather than thinking of status simply as the cultural dimension of class (Bourdieu, 1984), this approach treats it as a distinct social mechanism through which we feel ourselves to be esteemed compared to the people around us whose opinion of us shapes our sense of who we are (Chan and Goldthorpe, 2007; Appiah, 2010). Our 'felt perceptions of rank' are at the heart of the status order, and they directly shape our sense of our own and other peoples' social worth (Turner, 1988: 4).

Status and emotions: pride and shame

We register our subjective perceptions of our status as emotions, whether in the form of pride in our ability to win the admiration of our peers, relief in managing to 'pass' as relatively competent in our social roles, or shame as we perceive that we have failed to measure up. Emotions such as anxiety, guilt, shame and embarrassment register negative evaluations of ourselves and our relative social status. As Taylor explains:

> in experiencing any one of these emotions the person concerned believes of herself that she has deviated from some norm and that in doing so she has altered her standing in the world. The self is the 'object' of these emotions, and what is believed amounts to an assessment of that self. (Taylor, 1985: 1)

Negative self-assessment operates through these emotions, and we may feel shame when our inability to meet certain normative expectations is exposed (Lewis, 1995). Shame involves a sense of unintentional self-exposure that is experienced in embodied ways, either through blushing or some other physical indicator of one's dishonour (Lynd, 1958). Williams argues that shame is imagined in terms of nakedness and sexual exposure, which involves uncontrolled and improper revelations, and a desire to disappear (Williams, 1993). However, shame isn't only the feeling of being discovered displaying our actual or symbolic 'nakedness': we can also experience shame by imagining such discovery, and feel diminished in our own eyes as a result. Shame focuses on what we feel that we are, while guilt focuses our attention on what we have done to others and calls for some form of reparation. This means that we can feel both guilt and shame about the same action. Guilt focuses on others rather than on the self, whereas shame focuses on the self, which provides us with some understanding of who we seem to be, how we relate to others and how this fits with what we hope to be; it allows the possibility that we might be able to recreate ourselves as a result (Williams, 1993: 93).

Because of this quality, shame has been described as the 'premier' social emotion in evaluating the relationship between the self and wider social and moral norms. The experience of shame, or fear of shame, indicates our perception that we may lose all esteem, be cut adrift and no longer entitled to a position in the social order (Scheff, 2000). Our sensitivities to the subtle dynamics of social status lead to anxiety about the possibility of shame, and our constant anticipation of it motivates our actions. This may explain why people who are routinely and objectively considered to be of low or negative status, such as women or racialised peoples, might try to transform their 'deeply discrediting attributes' (Goffman, 1963: 13) into less 'shameful' forms to claim some social esteem, for example, by lightening their skin tone (Scheff, 2000). In doing this, discredited agents recognise the norms which convey status, and paradoxically seek to claim that status by transforming their 'shameful' bodily features, however unsuccessfully (McBride, 2013).

Status anxiety, shame and breastfeeding

Mothers are confronted with these paradoxes of status as they face the problem of how best to nurture their babies in the early days and weeks following birth. The normative context of early mothering is highly complex and contested, and although high-quality infant care is defined in terms of maternal breastfeeding (Marshall et al, 2007; Wolf, 2007), the threat of shame from multiple sources is ever present (Murphy, 1999). The question of how to gain esteem for the quality of one's mothering is not at all straightforward (Phoenix et al, 1991; Warner, 2006; Smyth, 2012). Public debates about breastfeeding tend to include much broader tensions over expectations of femininity and female sexuality in motherhood (Carter, 1995), and the priority of 'natural' or scientific approaches to caregiving (Apple, 1987, 2006).

There is a conflict between expectations. On the one hand, there are Victorian gender norms around female sexual modesty (Carter, 1995). On the other hand, there are expectations that breastfeeding is the quality hallmark of early caregiving. This generates concerns that the distinction between the maternal and the sexual is at risk of breaking down in breastfeeding (Blum, 1999; Stearns, 1999; Earle, 2003). These anxieties resonate with Mary Douglas's well-known argument that efforts to maintain an ordered society, for example, by separating the sexual and the maternal, are often symbolised through fears of bodily 'pollution', especially the transfer of bodily fluids. She says, 'It is not difficult to see how pollution beliefs can be used in a dialogue of claims and counter-claims to status' (Douglas, 2002 [1966]:4). Anxieties about this tension in breastfeeding seem to be driven by this process, particularly among people with low or negative objective status who struggle to demonstrate their commitment to the social order.

Feminist debates have only recently addressed questions about the relationship between breastfeeding and gender equality. This reflects unease with breastfeeding based on the historic association with maternalism (Raphael, 1976), and the rival feminist political principle of women's choice (Van Esterik, 1994; Carter, 1995). Feminism did not previously regard feeding babies with infant formula as problematic because it makes some redistribution of domestic labour possible by allowing fathers to be involved in 'the more gratifying aspects of parenting' (Maher, 1992: 8) (see Chapter Six on nighttime feeding).

Early feminist work criticised the close relationship between manufacturers of infant formula and healthcare providers for the way this powerful alliance limited women's choices (Palmer, 1993). The more recent intensification of breastfeeding advocacy, and the take-up of Unicef's Baby Friendly Hospitals Initiative (WHO and Unicef, 1989; see 'UK policy context' in this volume), has weakened the power of providers of infant formula. Feminist attention has shifted towards considering whether and how breastfeeding promotion might itself have become a form of social control with which contemporary mothers must grapple (Knaak, 2010; Martin and Redshaw, 2011). Specific concerns are raised over the ways women at the lower reaches of the social gradient tend to be a target of advocacy work (see, for example, Carter, 1995: 20). Recent feminist work highlights the significance of carefully developed breastfeeding support for gender equality, and supporting sexual and intimate citizenship as an important dimension of women's autonomy and reproductive justice (Lister, 2002; Smyth, 2008; Smith, 2012; Stearns, 2013).

However, the moral expectations promoted in current breastfeeding advocacy face criticism (Knaak, 2010; Hausman et al, 2012). Taylor and Wallace argue that contemporary breastfeeding promotion tends to trigger shame rather than guilt in new mothers, with potentially destructive consequences (Taylor and Wallace, 2012b: 77). They argue that the shame provoked by breastfeeding campaigns is unlike the guilt which public health campaigns otherwise often rely on to change behaviour. Breastfeeding promotion tends to directly target the moral status of the embodied, gendered and sexualised self. Esteem is associated with breastfeeding mothers who 'successfully' put an intimate, sexualised and vulnerable body part to work for frequent caregiving. This sets a high standard for early motherhood at an already strained time, as new relationships are established, responsibilities taken on and care routines worked out.

Taylor and Wallace argue that women experience shame for not breastfeeding, or not breastfeeding enough, rather than guilt. Women who intend to breastfeed but for a whole variety of reasons find themselves unable to 'judge themselves as deficient: bad mothers, failures' (Taylor and Wallace, 2012b: 85). The rest of this chapter develops this analysis by exploring experiences of shame among women who participated in a study of early motherhood carried out in 2009–10 (see Smyth, 2012). This study aimed to examine how norms of selfhood shaped maternal experience across two sites in the UK and US (Northern Ireland and Southern California) rather than not breastfeeding specifically. Strong patterns of traditional values are evident in both sites, including belief in God, and respect for authority, nation and the patriarchal family. They differ in attitudes to diversity, equality and self-expression, with Northern Ireland having one of the lowest rates of toleration for diversity and support for self-expression in the English-speaking world (Inglehart and Baker, 2000). Consequently, these two sites were identified as potentially promising contexts for exploring complex patterns of role interpretation.

Twenty mothers, mostly middle class, were interviewed in each site. What follows focuses on the Northern Ireland subsample, so that the UK policy context can be more fully considered. Unprompted reflections on experiences with infant feeding and responses to pressure to breastfeed are examined below, guided by sociological literature on the moral, self-evaluative quality of shame. The analysis of anonymised interview material explores how unsolicited discussion of breastfeeding focused on feeling diminished in the eyes of significant others for breastfeeding in inappropriate places, not breastfeeding enough or not breastfeeding at all. Significant others included healthcare professionals, the women's male partners, their own mothers, friends and women in their families. The ways that women felt diminished in their own eyes is also discussed, as problems with establishing or sustaining breastfeeding meant that they saw themselves as having failed to become the mother they hoped they would be.

The pride and shame of infant feeding

'I was definitely, definitely proud of myself when I did all the breastfeeding and that. I definitely felt like I'd done a good thing. It wasn't easy, but I did it.' (Anita, British, middle-class, full-time mother)

Unsolicited explicit expressions of pride and positive self-evaluation at having established and sustained breastfeeding were commonly expressed in interviews. This demonstrated a clear understanding of the expectations of new mothers, and a feeling that they were performing well and entitled to feel good. Such feelings of pride were often hard won following difficulties, including the pain of cracked nipples and mastitis, and feeding when other people are present, whether visiting family members or strangers in more public places.

Shame about one's self as a mother was also commonly expressed when discussing feeding. For example, Elaine's health condition meant that she was advised not to breastfeed because to do so would have passed toxicity on to her baby. While she and her partner accepted this, she discovered that others did not:

> 'I felt quite isolated ... there was 40 of us in our class, it was a big, big group. And I was the only one [who wasn't planning to breastfeed], and I really felt the other mummies were looking at me. They probably weren't, but I, and I said to the midwife after, "Look, it's not that I don't want to, I can't!" And she said to me, "When the baby's born, some people give you advice then [about feeding with formula]," she said, "but we can't tell you now, because we have to be seen to promote breastfeeding." And I felt, and then, just silly things like, when we went to go to Boots [pharmacy], and we were buying [formula], you can't redeem [loyalty reward] points or anything against it. Because they promote breastfeeding.' (British, middle class, part-time employment)

Elaine found it difficult to accept the perception of negative reactions from other mothers, midwives and even from the pharmacy. By explaining that feeding her baby infant formula wasn't a choice but a necessity, she sought reassurance from the antenatal midwife that she wasn't falling below the standards expected of prospective mothers. This was not forthcoming, and she was left feeling the unexpected isolation of social disapproval for planning to feed her baby infant formula under any circumstances.

Rachel became very distressed when she realised that her health visitor judged that her early mothering wasn't going well:

> 'I injured my nipple. You know, it was extremely painful, very, very, very sore. And, I seen the health visitor ... once so, maybe with the advice from my mum and my friends, I stopped breastfeeding and ... expressed, three times a day and, gave her formula the rest of the time. So ... the health visitor came back ... 10 days later. And, there's no other words to describe it, she wasn't happy. ... I was left in tears. That was really the first time that I really cried, you know I thought that we were getting on well, and I was left to feel that, we weren't.' (British, upper-middle-class professional, full-time employment)

The distress Rachel recalls damaged her sense of herself as a competent mother, a shame response which is likely to cause withdrawal and isolation (Barbalet, 2001). Rachel did not return to breastfeeding after this – despite the continued insistence and disapproval of the health visitor involved – whispering, "I got through it."

Jennifer recalled the disapproval she experienced when she introduced a bottle of infant formula at night to her breastfed baby. She did this on the advice of a midwife who said that her baby would be more satisfied and content if she received a bottle of infant formula at night, and that their relationship could then improve:

'I went back to the breastfeeding support group the week after [introducing the bottle], another midwife [was there]. I ... told her I was doing this. [She] was obviously appalled and horrified that I stuck a bottle of formula in, as if I was giving the baby whiskey or something, you know, or like, knockout drops! So, it kind of made it feel, you know, I felt really guilty. And in a way, like I remember saying to one of my friends, who was also a breastfeeding mum, who had terrible trouble, it's almost easier to from the beginning say, "I'm not going to do it." Because then you don't get, kind of, you don't get that guilt trip whenever you talk about introducing one bottle. And I did like eight weeks exclusive, which was hard going 'cos Sarah fed, constantly. ... It's, "Why are you stopping?" not, "Well done, you did eight weeks, you had mastitis, you were exhausted, that was really tough. Sleepless nights, all the rest of it." It's like, "You should really continue, persevere, you should not give them formula," as if you're giving them something awful [laugh].' (British, middle-class, part-time employment)

Taylor and Wallace argue that when women refer to their feelings of guilt about breastfeeding, their emotional reactions are better described as shame, since they involve the feeling that they are not good mothers rather than that they have caused harm (Taylor and Wallace, 2012a). Jennifer's reflections seem to fit with this, since she didn't accept that feeding her baby infant formula was the equivalent of giving her baby whiskey. She introduced infant formula on the advice of a midwife, so didn't feel that she had caused harm to her baby. However, she did feel that the quality of her mothering was discredited in the breastfeeding support group, despite the effort she had gone to in persevering in the face of physical pain and sleep deprivation, and she was shocked that any modification in her feeding method would be enough to lose her hard-won early status as a good mother. Her response reflects her effort to protect herself from potential shame by withdrawing from those contexts where it may be experienced: her suggestion that it would have been better never to have exposed herself to such harsh judgement by not trying to breastfeed at all.

Women who were determined to breastfeed but found themselves unable to could go to some extremes to give their babies 'the best' early care. Zara, for example, struggled for months to feed her baby with expressed breast milk since he didn't cooperate with breastfeeding:

'I was so determined to breastfeed. You know I really wanted it, and when he was born, I had no milk. … He was a bit jaundiced and, we just had to give him a bottle because he was hungry. I had no milk. And then, once you do that, [there's no going back]. I really thought I could, you know, whenever we come back, you know, [to our] home environment, it will be easier to happen. We really really tried for weeks. And, no, he would just cry every time he was put on the breast. He just wouldn't take it, so. I was very very disappointed. There was midwives that come out to the house, you know every day, they were all coming and, every day we were trying, different positions and, you know. So I was very very disappointed 'cos you want the best for them, and breast milk is the best, but, I couldn't. I started, pumping. And then, then it made everything, more, harder, because you're pumping and you are feeding so it's like doubling the work. So it was very very stressful because I had to get up every morning earlier than he did. Come down, pump for half an hour and then he woke up, and then, you know, it was just very stressful. And all day, because he was such a handful, I was stressing about not being able to pump and … [worried that] my milk will dry up and, you know. And then once he went down [to sleep], I had to pump again in the evening …, it was very very, you know, stressful and, I was doing it for three months.

I remember I went to a baby massage [class] with him and, everyone was breastfeeding and, and no one had the dummy and, everyone's baby was happy and, I just felt like such a failure, you know?' (Eastern European, middle-class, full-time employment)

A woman's feelings of shame at not being the mother she had hoped to become could be overwhelming. Ciara, a healthcare professional, broke down recalling her feelings about not being able to breastfeed her infant son:

> 'I wanted to breastfeed, and couldn't. It was just, he didn't latch on properly, but I kept insisting and insisting. I wanted to give this a go, and he was crying. There was one day, … he was on my breast for 23 hours. And he was trying to feed. He was trying and trying. And he just wasn't getting enough. So then, we did start bottle feeding. After about three weeks, I kept going and kept going for about three weeks, but every time I was putting him on I was in agony. So I kept thinking, I'm not doing this right, I'm a terrible mother. (Irish, lower middle-class, part-time employment)

This sense of shame was difficult to cope with, and Ciara commented that she felt she needed counselling to come to terms with not breastfeeding. A lone parent, her self-isolation reflected her deep sense of shame:

> 'I think I just sort of wanted to cocoon myself with him, and just have everybody, like, go away, either pre-empt what I need and do it for me directly or just don't bother even coming at all because, you know, I just can't handle it.'

This illustrates Lynd's argument that 'the experience of shame is itself isolating, alienating, incommunicable' (1958: 67). Ciara's sense of herself as a good mother improved, however, as she watched her son thrive following the introduction of infant formula, as well as due to the reassurance she received from her own mother throughout this time.

Conclusion

Infant feeding is often experienced as emotionally intense, not only because of practical concerns with how one's baby might be growing and thriving, but also because of the moralised approach to promotion strategies. When breastfeeding is established as the hallmark of good mothering, the feeling that one is failing can be very damaging, whether one is not breastfeeding at all, not breastfeeding appropriately or not breastfeeding with sufficient dedication. It should be no surprise that advertising for infant formula explicitly reassures non-breastfeeding mothers that this approach to feeding also signals devotion to infant health, bonding and taking pride in children's development (Aptamil, 2016).

Taylor and Wallace argue that the shaming effects of current breastfeeding advocacy also undermine attempts to normalise the practice, as avoiding potential shame can mean avoiding breastfeeding completely (Taylor and Wallace, 2012b). Louise, an upper-middle-class full-time mother, recalled that during her second pregnancy, 'I just said [to midwives], "Right guys, just don't even talk to me about it. I'm not doing it."' It should be no surprise that those much lower down on the social gradient than Louise are most reluctant to risk their feelings about themselves as good, esteem-worthy mothers, and avoid breastfeeding completely.

The question of how best to facilitate breastfeeding without threatening new mothers' fragile self-evaluations and status is an urgent one for health policy. Rather than simple slogans and solutions, a more nuanced, less moralised approach is necessary. This should focus on the structures within which early mothering takes place, not on individual women and their partners.

References

Appiah, A. (2010) *The honor code: how moral revolutions happen*, New York: W. W. Norton.

Apple, R. D. (1987) *Mothers and medicine: A social history of infant feeding, 1890–1950*, Madison, WI: University of Wisconsin Press.

Apple, R. D. (2006) *Perfect motherhood: Science and childrearing in America*, New Brunswick, NJ: Rutgers University Press.

Aptamil (2016) 'Aptamil follow on milk – today for tomorrow', www.youtube.com/watch?v=OH1WUV39sAc

Barbalet, J. M. (2001) *Emotion, social theory and social structure: A macrosociological approach*, Cambridge: Cambridge University Press.

Benard, S. and Correll, S. J. (2010) 'Normative discrimination and the motherhood penalty', *Gender and Society*, 24(5): 616–46.

Blair-Loy, M. (2003) *Competing devotions: Career and family among women executives*, Cambridge, MA: Harvard University Press.

Blum, L. M. (1999) *At the breast: Ideologies of breastfeeding and motherhood in the contemporary United States*, Boston, MA: Beacon Press.

Bourdieu, P. (1984) *Distinction: A social critique of the judgement of taste*, Cambridge, MA: Harvard University Press.

Brennan, G. and Pettit, P. (2004) *The economy of esteem: An essay on civil and political society*, Oxford: Oxford University Press.

Callaghan, J.E.M. and Lazard, L. (2011) "'Please don't put the whole dang thing out there!": a discursive analysis of internet discussions around infant feeding', *Psychology and Health*, 27(8): 938–55.

Carter, P. (1995) *Feminism, breasts and breast-feeding*, Basingstoke: Macmillan Press Ltd.

Chan, T. W. and Goldthorpe, J. H. (2007) 'Class and status: the conceptual distinction and its empirical relevance', *American Sociological Review*, 72(4): 512–32.

Chuang, C.-H., Chang, P.-J., Chen, Y.-C., Hsieh, W.-S., Hurng, B.-S., Lin, S.-J.and Chen, P.-C. (2010) 'Maternal return to work and breastfeeding: a population-based cohort study', *International Journal of Nursing Studies*, 47(4): 461–74.

Douglas, M. (2002 [1966]) *Purity and danger: An analysis of concepts of pollution and taboo*, London: Routledge.

Dowling, S., Naidoo, J. and Pontin, D. (2012) 'Breastfeeding in public: women's bodies, women's milk', in P. H. Smith, B. L. Hausman and M. Labbok (eds) *Beyond health, beyond choice: Breastfeeding constraints and realities*, New Brunswick, NJ: Rutgers University Press, pp 249–58.

Dykes, F. and Flacking, R. (2010) 'Encouraging breastfeeding: a relational perspective', *Early Human Development*, 86(11): 733–6.

Earle, S. (2003) 'Is breast best? breastfeeding, motherhood and identity', in S. Earle and G. Letherby (eds) *Gender, identity and reproduction: Social perspectives*, Basingstoke: Palgrave Macmillan, pp 135–50.

Frank, R. H. (2007) *Falling behind: How rising inequality harms the middle class*, Berkeley, CA: University of California Press.

Goffman, E. (1951) 'Symbols of class status', *British Journal of Sociology*, 2(4): 294–304.

Goffman, E. (1963) *Stigma: Notes on the management of spoiled identity*, Englewood Cliffs, NJ: Prentice-Hall.

Goffman, E. (1971 [1956]) *The presentation of self in everyday life*, Harmondsworth: Penguin.

Hausman, B. L., Smith, P. H. and Labbok, M. H. (2012) 'Introduction: breastfeeding constraints and realities', in P. H. Smith, B. L. Hausman and M. Labbok (eds) *Beyond health, beyond choice: Breastfeeding constraints and realities*, New Brunswick, NJ: Rutgers University Press, pp 1–11.

Hinde, K. (2017) 'What we don't know about mother's milk', in B. Warburg (ed) *TED Talks*, https://www.ted.com/talks/katie_hinde_what_we_don_t_know_about_mother_s_milk

Inglehart, R. and Baker, W. E. (2000) 'Modernization, cultural change, and the persistence of traditional values', *American Sociological Review*, 65(1): 19–51.

Kelleher, C. M. (2006) 'The physical challenges of early breastfeeding', *Social Science and Medicine*, 63(10): 2727–38.

Knaak, S. J. (2010) 'Contextualising risk, constructing choice: breastfeeding and good mothering in risk society', *Health, Risk and Society*, 12(4), 345–55.

Lewis, M. (1995) *Shame: The exposed self*, New York: Free Press.

Lewis, J., Knijn, T., Martin, C. and Ostner, I. (2008) 'Patterns of development in work/family reconciliation policies for parents in France, Germany, the Netherlands, and the UK in the 2000s', *Social Politics: International Studies in Gender, State and Society*, 15(3): 261–86.

Lister, R. (2002) 'Sexual citizenship', in E. F. Isin and B. S. Turner (eds) *Handbook of citizenship studies*, London: Sage, pp 191–207.

Lynd, H. M. (1958) *On shame and the search for identity*, New York: Harcourt, Brace and Company.

Maher, V. (1992) 'Breast-feeding in cross-cultural perspective: paradoxes and proposals', in V. Maher (ed) *The anthropology of breast-feeding: natural law or social construct*, Oxford: Berg, pp. 1–36.

Marshall, J. L., Godfrey, M. and Renfrew, M. J. (2007) 'Being a "good mother": managing breastfeeding and merging identities', *Social Science and Medicine*, 65(10): 2147–59.

Martin, C. R. and Redshaw, M. (2011) 'Is breast always best? balancing benefits and choice?', *Journal of Reproductive and Infant Psychology*, 29(2): 113–14.

McAndrew, F., Thompson, J., Fellows, L., Large, A., Speed, M. and Renfrew, M. J. (2012) 'Infant Feeding Survey 2010', https://digital.nhs.uk/catalogue/PUB08694

McBride, C. (2013) *Recognition*, Cambridge: Polity Press.

Miracle, D. J. and Fredland, V. (2007) 'Provider encouragement of breastfeeding: efficacy and ethics', *Journal of Midwifery and Women's Health*, 52(6): 545–8.

Murphy, E. (1999) '"Breast is best": infant feeding decisions and maternal deviance', *Sociology of Health and Illness*, 21(2): 187–208.

Palmer, G. (1993) *The politics of breastfeeding*, London: Pandora.

Phoenix, A., Woollett, A. and Lloyd, E. (1991) *Motherhood: Meanings, practices and ideologies*, London: Sage.

Raphael, D. (1976) *The tender gift: Breastfeeding*, New York: Schocken Books.

Ridgeway, C. L. and Correll, S. J. (2004) 'Motherhood as a status characteristic', *Journal of Social Issues*, 60(4): 683–700.

Ryan, K., Smith, L. and Alexander, J. (2013) 'When baby's chronic illness and disability interfere with breastfeeding: women's emotional adjustment', *Midwifery*, 29(7): 794–800.

Scheff, T. J. (2000) 'Shame and the social bond: a sociological theory', *Sociological Theory*, 18(1): 84–99.

Smith, P. H. (2012) 'Breastfeeding promotion through gender equity: a theoretical perspective for public health practice', in P. H. Smith, B. L. Hausman and M. Labbok (eds) *Beyond health, beyond choice: Breastfeeding constraints and realities*, New Brunswick, NJ: Rutgers University Press, pp 25–35.

Smyth, L. (2008) 'Gendered spaces and intimate citizenship', *European Journal of Women's Studies*, 15(2): 83–99.

Smyth, L. (2012) *The demands of motherhood: agents, roles and recognition*, Basingstoke: Palgrave Macmillan.

Stearns, C. (1999) 'Breastfeeding and the good maternal body', *Gender and Society*, 13(3) 308–325.

Stearns, C. (2013) 'The embodied practices of breastfeeding: implications for research and policy', *Journal of Women, Politics and Policy*, 34(4): 359–70.

Stewart, F. H. (1994) *Honor*, Chicago, IL: University of Chicago Press.

Strong, G. (2013) 'Barriers to breastfeeding during the neonatal period', *Journal of Neonatal Nursing*, 19(4), 134–8.

Sunstein, C. R. (1996) 'Social norms and social roles', *Columbia Law Review*, 96(4): 903–68.

Taylor, G. (1985) *Pride, shame, and guilt: Emotions of self-assessment*, Oxford: Clarendon Press.

Taylor, E. N. and Wallace, L. E. (2012a) 'Feminist breastfeeding promotion and the problem of guilt', in P. H. Smith, B. L. Hausman and M. Labbok (eds) *Beyond health, beyond choice: Breastfeeding constraints and realities*, New Brunswick, NJ: Rutgers University Press, pp 193–202

Taylor, E. N. and Wallace, L. E. (2012b) 'For shame: feminism, breastfeeding advocacy and maternal guilt', *Hypatia*, 27(1): 76–98.

Thompson, R. E., Kildea, S. V., Barclay, L. M. and Kruske, S. (2011) 'An account of significant events influencing Australian breastfeeding practice over the last 40 years', *Women and Birth*, 24(3): 97–104.

Turner, B. S. (1988) *Status*, Milton Keynes: Open University Press.

Van Esterik, P. (1994) 'Breastfeeding and feminism', *International Journal of Gynecology and Obstetrics*, 47 (suppl.): 41–54.

Van Wagenen, S. A., Magnusson, B. M. and Neiger, B. (2015) 'Attitudes toward breastfeeding among an internet panel of US males aged 21–44', *Maternal and Child Health Journal*, 19(9): 2020–28.

Victora, C. G., Bahl, R., Barros, A.J.D., França, G.V.A., Horton, S., Krasevec, J., Murch, S., Sankar, M. J., Walker, N. and Rollins, N. C., on behalf of the Lancet Breastfeeding Series Group (2016) 'Breastfeeding in the 21st century: epidemiology, mechanisms, and lifelong effect', *The Lancet*, 387(10017): 475–90.

Wambach, K. A. and Cohen, S. M. (2009) 'Breastfeeding experiences of urban adolescent mothers', *Journal of Pediatric Nursing*, 24(4): 244–54.

Warner, J. (2006) *Perfect madness: Motherhood in the age of anxiety*, London: Vermilion.

Weber, M. (1978) *Economy and society: An outline of interpretive sociology*, Berkeley, CA: University of California Press.

Williams, B. (1993) *Shame and necessity*, Berkeley, CA: University of California Press.

Wolf, J. B. (2007) 'Is breast really best? risk and total motherhood in the national breastfeeding awareness campaign', *Journal of Health Politics, Policy and Law*, 32(4): 595–636.

World Health Organization (2003) *Global strategy for infant and child feeding*, Geneva: WHO.

World Health Organization and Unicef (1989) *Protecting, promoting and supporting breast-feeding: The special role of maternity services*, Geneva: WHO.

THREE

'Betwixt and between': women's experiences of breastfeeding long term

Sally Dowling

Introduction

This chapter draws on my research with women who breastfeed for longer than is usual in the UK, where a minority of women are still breastfeeding at six months and an unknown number breastfeed into the second year of life and beyond (McAndrew et al, 2012). The anthropological concept of liminality (being 'neither one thing nor another') is used to explore and understand their experiences. The chapter takes ideas about liminality and relates them to breastfeeding long term, discussing how they might help those working in this area to support more mothers to breastfeed for longer. It briefly outlines what is known about long-term breastfeeding from previous research and explains the concept of liminality.

The remainder of the chapter discusses the findings in relation to liminality and how this has been used to think about breastfeeding, and considers what being 'betwixt and between' means for breastfeeding women. The idea of breastfeeding as polluting or 'matter out of place' (Douglas, 2002 [1966]) is also briefly discussed. The research project contributes to other publications (Dowling and Brown, 2013; Tomori et al, 2016; Dowling and Pontin, 2017) but this chapter focuses on how it might be used in breastfeeding support both in a wider, cultural sense, and by healthcare practitioners and volunteers.

Background

What do we know about long-term breastfeeding and health?

The focus in this chapter is on social and cultural experiences of breastfeeding long term, rather than physical health. The health consequences of *not* breastfeeding are well established, and there are known problems in carrying out research in this area: ethical difficulties with randomised controlled trials (RCTs) lead to a dependence on observational and cohort studies (Horta and Victora, 2013). Despite these difficulties, the evidence in relation to breastfeeding recommendations is stronger than ever (Victora et al, 2016). Carrying out research on long-term breastfeeding is particularly difficult, as sample sizes are small and older breastfeeders have many other influences on their health. However, there is a known dose–response relationship for many of the health consequences of having been breastfed; that is, the more breast milk a baby receives the greater the influence on health or protection against illness. Breastfeeding for longer periods is therefore recognised as important in having a positive effect on childhood mortality and morbidity, lifelong health conditions and women's health (Victora et al, 2016).

What do we know about the experience of long-term breastfeeding?

Most of the academic work on the experience of long-term breastfeeding is from the US, Canada and Australia, and although it is now dated (see, for example, Morse and Harrison, 1987; Reamer and Sugarman, 1987; Hills-Bonczyk et al, 1994), recent publications (including Rempel, 2004; Gribble, 2007; Gribble, 2008; and Stearns, 2011) have similar findings. Women who breastfeed long term talk about others' perception that they are carrying out a socially unacceptable/inappropriate practice (Stearns, 2011). This can lead them to hide their continued breastfeeding, sometimes from their family and friends, and often from healthcare professionals (Buckley, 2001; Rempel, 2004; Gribble, 2007, 2008). Support may be withdrawn as time goes on (particularly after 12 months), which is experienced as pressure to wean. Mothers often report comments like, "Are you still nursing?" or, "Why are you still doing that?" at the end of the first year (Dowling and Brown, 2013). Women who breastfeed long term value the support they gain from organisations such as La Leche League (LLL), where long-term breastfeeding is normalised (Stearns, 2011) and 'expected' (Gribble, 2008: 12), and women's decisions are validated (Faircloth, 2010a).

Recent research has looked at long-term breastfeeding in the UK. This includes the study drawn on in this chapter (see also Dowling and Brown, 2013; Tomori et al, 2016; Dowling and Pontin, 2017) and Faircloth's work (for example, 2010a, 2010b, 2011). Interviews for the UK health experiences website healthtalk.org also include experiences of breastfeeding long term. These were carried out in 2005–06 and are drawn on in other work, for example, Ryan, Todres and Alexander (2011). Faircloth associates long-term breastfeeding with maternal identity, and how mothers make sense of their decisions which are different to those made by most other women; she also writes about the relationship between long-term breastfeeding and attachment parenting (Sears and Sears, 2001). The healthtalk.org interviews echo experiences written about in the literature, including the way initial approval for breastfeeding changes to disapproval, the fact that longer-term breastfeeding is more likely to be done in private, and the importance of support from a range of people and from groups.

A recently published concept analysis of long-term breastfeeding considered how nurses could 'support and promote breastfeeding beyond infancy' (Brockway and Venturato, 2016: 2004). Published literature was reviewed and characteristics essential to longer-term breastfeeding – health benefits, maternal profiles, parenting style and experiences – were identified, – along with consequences, which included stigma and secrecy. Some of the US and UK work discussed in this chapter was included in this analysis and the findings resonate with the study findings discussed here.

Breastfeeding for longer than the norm is described here as 'long-term breastfeeding'. It is referred to in a variety of ways in the literature, media, and in discussions online and between mothers and their supporters, including 'extended', 'full-term' and 'sustained' breastfeeding. One interesting finding from the study discussed in this chapter is that, when asked, women who were breastfeeding long term had no word to describe what they did – perhaps demonstrating their status as being between social identities.

What does 'liminality' mean and how is it useful?

Liminality is a concept from anthropology used to think about rites of passage – the ways people move from being in one life stage to another and their associated rituals. It is most associated with Van Gennep (1960 [1909]), whose work was later developed by Turner (2009 [1969]). The word 'liminality' comes from the Latin *limen*, meaning threshold. Liminality usually refers to the idea of being 'betwixt and between' (Turner, 2009 [1969]), neither one thing nor another. It is the phase when the old life is left behind but the new way of being has not yet started, a time when a person is neither how they were previously nor how they will be in the future. Van Gennep associated different phases with this: 'separation' (the pre-liminal phase, when people move from their previous life), 'transition' (the liminal phase, when they are neither how they were before nor how they will be afterwards), and 'incorporation' (the post-liminal time, when a person comes back into society, socially different to how they were before). Modern day rites of passage include, for example, getting married, leaving home, graduating from university and becoming a parent.

Liminality is also written about in relation to ideas of pollution, danger and social discomfort (Douglas, 2002 [1966]). People in a liminal phase are ambiguous, separate and sometimes seen as threatening. Douglas wrote about how bodily fluids (such as menstrual fluids) are perceived as 'matter out of place' when separated from the body (see also Chapter Two); I also apply these ideas here to breast milk (as do Mahon-Daly and Andrews, 2002). When people are together in a liminal phase, they have been described as occupying a common space, called 'communitas' (Turner, 2009 [1969]). This refers to a way of living, rather than an actual place (Madge and O'Connor, 2005); it is not so much about identity but a common experience, 'a shared sense of alterity' (Czarniawska and Mazza, 2003: 273; quoted in Dowling and Pontin, 2017: 60). This is further discussed later in the chapter.

Liminality has been adapted, developed and used to think about a range of issues, including health. More recent ways of writing about it do not always identify clearly the three stages outlined above; the focus is often on the 'betwixt and between' nature of the experience. Recent examples include using liminality to think about parents' experiences of caring for a dying child (Jordan et al, 2015), living with a life-threatening illness (Bruce et al, 2014) and undergoing late-stage cancer therapy (Adorno, 2015). It has been used specifically to think about women's health issues, for example, the biographical disruption caused by treatment for early-stage breast cancer (Trusson et al, 2016), experiences of fertility and fertility clinics (Allen, 2007) and how women make decisions about seeking help after discovering a breast symptom (Granek and Fergus, 2012). Sometimes the transition to the liminal state is unintended and this may exacerbate the powerlessness; the change may also be invisible to others, for example, having an abnormal cervical smear (Forss et al, 2004) (see Dowling and Pontin (2017) for further examples and discussion).

As a concept, liminality has not been used much to think in detail about breastfeeding, although it has been referred to (see, for example, Groleau et al, 2006; Sachs et al, 2006; Dykes, 2009; Boyer, 2011). Recently, Shattnawi (2015) has written about breastfeeding in neonatal intensive care (NICU) as a liminal experience, where women find their rite of passage to becoming a mother disrupted.

Mahon-Daly and Andrews' (2002) work is important here, although it is dated and doesn't mention long-term breastfeeding. They were the only researchers using liminality as a central concept to think about breastfeeding experiences in relation to space, place and rites of passage until the study discussed here.

Mahon-Daly and Andrews rework the original concept, focusing in particular on the transitional stage, discussing breastfeeding and liminality in relation to three 'levels' (2002: 65). In this chapter, findings from my research study are discussed in relation to these three levels because of the importance of this earlier work. Mahon-Daly and Andrews' ideas about breastfeeding and liminality are used to illuminate the experience of women who breastfeed long-term. These three levels are:

1. The postnatal period;
2. The ways in which breastfeeding changes women for life;
3. Breastfeeding itself, particularly the ways in which women behave in different places while breastfeeding.

In the third level, rituals are considered, relating this to the more traditional explanations of the transition phase of liminality. Mahon-Daly and Andrews consider breastfeeding as a liminal activity in relation to time and space; and they refer to the perceived impurity/dirtiness of breast milk by the women in their study – relating this to Douglas's (2002 [1966]) ideas – reinforcing the liminal nature of breastfeeding. Central to their explanation is the idea that breastfeeding is not a 'normal' activity, and that women want to return to a 'normal' life. This may be the experience of many women, but it raises issues for creating social and cultural support for breastfeeding in order to normalise it at all ages and in all settings, which is a central theme of recent research (Rollins et al, 2016) and campaigns (Unicef, 2016).

Methods used in the study

The remainder of this chapter's discussion draws on a research study for which data was collected between 2008 and 2010. Three qualitative methods – participant observation, and face-to-face (FTF) and email interviews – were used to find out more about the experience of breastfeeding long term. I was also a long-term breastfeeder at this time, and so conducted the research from an 'insider' perspective (Dowling, 2009). For the purposes of the study, and in the context of poor UK breastfeeding rates, 'long-term' was defined as longer than six months.

Participant observation enabled contact with over 80 mothers in three breastfeeding support groups in different areas of a large UK city, one an LLL group and two in more socially diverse areas. These mothers were breastfeeding newborns to four-year-olds. Interviews were with 10 mothers (six face-to-face, four via email). Between them they had breastfed/were breastfeeding 15 children up to six and a half years old. Their experiences included breastfeeding while pregnant and tandem feeding, and some had breastfed continuously for many years. Notes were taken during or after support group meetings, FTF interviews were transcribed in full and email interviews were imported into Microsoft Word. All data was analysed thematically (Braun and Clarke, 2006) as well as in relation to theoretical concepts of stigma, taboo and liminality. These methods are detailed elsewhere (see Dowling, 2011; Dowling and Pontin, 2017). All names are pseudonyms and the University of the West of England, Bristol, granted ethical approval for the study.

Discussion: women's experiences of breastfeeding long term

Four main themes capture the women's discussion of their experiences: deciding to breastfeed long term, commitment (living with long-term breastfeeding), challenges in breastfeeding long term, and being supported in long-term breastfeeding (discussed in more detail in Dowling and Pontin, 2017). The overall impression was of a group of very strong-willed and determined women. The mothers made choices in relation to breastfeeding and parenting that, although they felt right for their child/children, led to some personal hardship and isolation, and were sometimes experienced as very challenging. Many participants talked about a range of other parenting decisions they made in relation to long-term breastfeeding, which are also discussed in the literature: attachment parenting – including sling-wearing and co-sleeping – and home-educating (see, for example, Faircloth, 2010a, 2010b). These themes are considered here in relation to how they illustrate the liminal nature of the experience of long-term breastfeeding, broadly using the schema proposed by Mahon-Daly and Andrews. These are reinterpreted here as 'the postnatal phase and beyond', 'being changed by breastfeeding', and 'using people and places to support breastfeeding'; under these headings the main themes of this study are discussed.

Most mothers planned to breastfeed, talking about this in relation to 'always knowing' that they would, their knowledge of the health and other benefits, the influence of other people, and the feeling that they had 'no choice'/'it's natural'. Few intended to breastfeed long term, describing it as something that just happened gradually once breastfeeding was established:

'I think a lot of long-term breastfeeders are the same … they [don't] necessarily have a goal, "I'm going to feed until they're two," … often it's just a gradual thing that happens.' (Josie)

'I don't think I thought, "I am going to breastfeed for a long time," I just thought I'll see how it goes really.' (Jane)

Some felt that as health promotion messages mentioned six months in relation to breastfeeding, this was a suggested cut-off (although in fact it refers to exclusive breastfeeding duration and not overall duration, discussed further in Dowling and Brown, 2013):

'It didn't really occur to me to think about when I end … I just assumed there must be a time everyone stops … I never knew what that age was, I suppose either six months or twelve.' (Sam)

'I wanted to do the … national six months recommendation … I wanted to do six months…' (Josie)

Most mothers had never seen an older baby or child breastfeeding before they breastfed themselves; those that had seen it described the experience as 'surprising', 'shocking' (Dowling and Pontin, 2017) or odd:

'I'd often felt uncomfortable at the idea of feeding older babies and toddlers … I might have sort of gone, "Oh that looks a bit odd."' (Jane)

Most did not think it was something they would do, but as time went on did not want to stop. They enjoyed breastfeeding and felt it was right for them and their child to continue. For some this became related to other parenting decisions and a desire to be led by the child; it was a 'gift' – "I think really it's this amazing gift I've given [son]. I just don't think I'll be able to come close to doing anything as good for him ever again" (Tina) – and an important parenting tool – "I like the way it solved so many problems" (Christine).

The postnatal phase and beyond

In Mahon-Daly and Andrews' discussion of breastfeeding and liminality, the first liminal phase is the postnatal one. Women who breastfeed, by being neither 'pregnant' nor 'not pregnant', are not reintegrated into society straight away, and so transition is not immediately experienced. Women who are breastfeeding are different to other women: 'Breastfeeding bodies are physically different ... relatively uncommon ... experienced by a minority'(Mahon-Daly and Andrews, 2002: 65). Women who breastfeed for a long time or for longer than the norm have an experience which continues to be different both to those who have stopped breastfeeding and to those who have never breastfed. In this phase, women do not know what they or their future will be like.

In my study, mothers talked about many ways in which they felt different. They talked about how they felt they were in a phase that it was hard to see an end to, in relation to having another child, returning to paid work or other ways in which they would feel 'back to normal'. Mothers talked about being extremely tired – "It was exhausting" (Sarah); "I just remember being so exhausted" (Tina) – feeling "touched out, I'd love to have some *space*," (woman in LLL group); "I so much longed for a night without her climbing on me" (Sarah); and lonely. Those who used the principles of attachment parenting particularly felt that they were in a place from which it was hard to move; for many this was part of the commitment they had made to their child, and long-term breastfeeding was an element of this.

Participants made decisions about many aspects of caring for and breastfeeding their children which they felt set them apart from other mothers. They gave examples of how they saw themselves as being in a different place than that they had been in before they became mothers, in relation to breastfeeding as well as to other aspects of parenting. These included where the baby slept, whether they were carried in a sling for long periods, how often and for how long they breastfed, and for some later, how they were educated. Many families chose to co-sleep but found it very difficult when it had an impact on their rest, relationships and intimacy with partners. The women's loneliness was exacerbated by knowledge that they were different from other families around them. For many this was emotionally and physically isolating – a 'cost' (Sarah). Sarah also talked about the commitment that was made to a way of life, a phase that 'continues without a clear end in sight'.

This commitment to a way of life places women in a liminal space – both because of the decisions that they make and because of the way they are seen by society. Women who do not conform to expectations and norms are transgressive: 'breastfeeding can be constructed as a refusal of the woman to make the expected rite of passage back to the pre-pregnant state, extending a dangerous or liminal state'(Smale, 2001: 240). Feeling different was also reinforced by comments from others, particularly grandparents and some fathers who felt that their relationship with the child was constrained because of continued breastfeeding.

Being changed by breastfeeding

In Mahon-Daly and Andrews' second stage, breastfeeding changes women and their understandings of themselves and their bodies, a 'new world' (Mahon-Daly and Andrews, 2010: 65) which is communicated to other people. Mothers in my study talked about many ways in which they felt they had been changed by breastfeeding, as well as how they talked about this with others. This was in relation to what they did, but also to how this was enabled. They talked about their qualities of determination and confidence – "I'm very clear in my mind that I'm doing the best for my baby so I don't mind what other people think" (Lucia) – and how they prevented others from criticising them – "Perhaps my ... assumption that no one would object meant that all were intimidated into not doing so!" (Jess). They also expressed how much pleasure they gained from breastfeeding – "I love this! I don't want it to stop!" (woman at an LLL observation) – and the closeness/ bond it gave them with their child.

For many, being changed by breastfeeding went together with being challenged by it. Breastfeeding in public was one specific challenge (discussed in the next section in relation to the use of place). Many participants talked about how they had internalised expectations about what would be acceptable, and anticipated negative reactions from others even if they were not forthcoming. They talked about waiting for negative comments, and being surprised when nothing was said, but nonetheless often felt "awkward" (Sam), "very uncomfortable" (Josie) or "self-conscious" (Judith).

Mothers in this study talked about longer-term breastfeeding in ways that illustrate the idea of 'matter out of place', discussed earlier in the chapter. They talked about places and situations where they understood that their breast milk was not expected/acceptable as the child grew older – in church, for example, and in public places. They talked about when and where breastfeeding and their lactating breasts felt comfortable and when they didn't – referring, for example, to feeling "on display" (Josie). The actions of women who breastfeed long term place them in a liminal state and make both their bodies and their breast milk 'matter out of place', reinforcing taboos. In many social situations, breast milk is a taboo body fluid, and the women in this study illustrate this with examples of where breastfeeding wasn't comfortable. Stearns has also written about this in relation to breastfeeding children who 'walk, talk and take' (2011: 547).

Being open about doing something that is interpreted as culturally transgressive provokes stigmatising reactions from others (Smale, 2001; Tomori et al, 2016). Liminal states can be perceived as disturbing; liminal people as ambiguous and separate. Women who continue to breastfeed longer than is culturally normal demonstrate the cultural unacceptability of a liminal state with no apparent end. Women who carry on breastfeeding beyond infancy experience pressure to wean. Mothers in my study were asked, "Why are you still breastfeeding?" (woman at LLL meeting). They said that, "People express surprise if you are breastfeeding longer than a year, like you are a funny person" (woman at LLL meeting), or that, "They just assume that I've stopped" (woman at LLL meeting, with an 18-month-old). These women recognised that they were choosing to behave in a way that set them apart from others.

Using places and people to support breastfeeding

The final stage in Mahon-Daly and Andrews' explanation talks about the places and spaces breastfeeding women use to ensure comfort when breastfeeding. The mothers in my study talked a lot about the use of space in relation to breastfeeding in public – sometimes interpreting spaces as public or private according to who they were with. Home could be private but also public, even when breastfeeding in front of family, particularly as the child grew older. Women with older toddlers breastfed in public places, and nearly all said they were comfortable doing this. However, they described strategies they used to make it easier, such as not making eye contact with strangers – "I just don't meet people's eyes" (Jess) – not breastfeeding alone, using a corner of the room or turning their back on others – "I just kind of ignore people around me, when I'm doing it (Sam). These are strategies also described in the literature in relation to breastfeeding at any age (see, for example, Stearns, 1999, 2011).

Groups were spaces used both to breastfeed and to discuss it. They were particularly valued for the opportunities they offered for talking about long-term breastfeeding and related behaviours, such as tandem nursing, breastfeeding while pregnant and co-sleeping. For some mothers, there was also a gradual association with other groups, such as for home education support. Mothers gravitated towards places and people that made them feel comfortable. These are subcultures, enabling women through their support to remain in a liminal space for some time and with some security. Several women did not move back (reincorporate) into society in the way that they had previously been, but came to identify themselves after a period of being 'betwixt and between' in a new and different way, as attachment parents or home educators or birth supporters/doulas. For other mothers, the liminal phase was clearer and there was an intention to return to life as it was before.

The clear feeling of belonging to a community that was experienced by some mothers is an example of 'communitas'. This was not true for all participants but for many, particularly LLL attendees and those who labelled themselves as attachment parents, their identification as long-term breastfeeders and with other women who had made similar parenting decisions gave them the shared sense of belonging to a community, as identified by Czarniawksa and Mazza (2003). Some women talked specifically about how this shared community did not need a physical presence and how it could be online or found through reading books and accounts of others' experiences.

Mothers in this study also talked about other people who supported them, and those who were unhelpful. Partners were usually supportive, other family members less so, particularly mothers and mothers-in-law. Health professionals were generally perceived as unhelpful and lacking in knowledge about continuing to breastfeed beyond infancy. Friends were often referred to as 'like-minded people' and were very important, particularly those who made similar breastfeeding and parenting choices. Many of the women described a dropping-off of contact with those women who had made other choices. Breastfeeding was sometimes hidden from those perceived or known to be unsupportive.

Conclusion: how does this help us to support women to breastfeed for longer?

There are several different interpretations of the idea of liminality that are built on the original anthropological understanding of the concept. Two main ways of thinking about liminality are important here: the 'rites of passage', when people experience ritualised transitions between states or life stages, and one with less clearly defined states. In this latter explanation, long-term breastfeeding is not one thing or another; it is ambiguous, 'seen as [a] "not quite either" or "some of both"' state (Jackson, 2005; quoted in Dowling and Pontin, 2017: 70). The related idea of 'matter out of place' is also of importance.

The study discussed here has furthered our understanding about what it is like to carry on breastfeeding when most other women have stopped. Drawing on the work of Mahon-Daly and Andrews (2002), and on other interpretations of liminality, it shows that women who breastfeed long term can find themselves in a liminal or 'betwixt and between' state, and continue to experience themselves as different, both from those who breastfed and have stopped and from those who never breastfed. Many of the women in this study found new interests, and for some new career directions that came from their experience of breastfeeding. This meant that they did not reincorporate into society as before, but were changed. Some women felt that the decisions they made about how they lived their lives and how they were as parents set them aside from others, particularly those women who called themselves attachment parents or who went on to home educate their children.

For some women who breastfeed, the liminal stage is a clear and temporary one. They eventually return to life as non-breastfeeding mothers, although changed forever by the experience of becoming and being a parent. For others, a new identity is forged through breastfeeding and there is recognition that things will not be the same again. This was particularly true in this study of women who identified themselves as long-term breastfeeders, perhaps breastfeeding for very long periods overall, with two or more children, or who became breastfeeding counsellors or doulas.

Recent reports and campaigns have highlighted the importance of social and cultural support for breastfeeding (Rollins et al, 2016; Unicef, 2016; McFadden et al, 2017). The stigma experienced by women who breastfeed beyond social norms, as well as those who carry out other, related breastfeeding and mothering practices, limits the amount and extent of support they receive (Tomori et al, 2016). One way we can begin to counter this is by accepting a range of breastfeeding durations as 'normal', including showing breastfeeding at many ages in health promotion materials (Dowling and Brown, 2013). Support for women who breastfeed their children at any age in public is also important both to destigmatise the practice and to normalise it; this is also true of support from health professionals and the wider community.

Theoretical ideas like liminality can help us to think about and understand women's experiences. However, without considering 'the complex interplay between individual, relationship, community and societal factors' (Labbok, 2012: 14) there is no framework in which to think about undertaking actions which could lead to change and greater support of women breastfeeding at all ages, and lead to increased continuation rates of breastfeeding in the UK.

References

Adorno, G. (2015) 'Between two worlds: liminality and late-stage cancer-directed therapy', *Omega: Journal of Death and Dying*, 71(2): 99–125.

Allen, H. (2007) 'Experiences of infertility: liminality and the role of the fertility clinic', *Nursing Inquiry*, 14: 132–9.

Boyer, K. (2011) '"The way to break the taboo is to do the taboo thing": lactation advocacy in the contemporary UK', *Health and Place*, 18(3): 430–37.

Braun, V. and Clarke, V. (2006) 'Using thematic analysis in psychology', *Qualitative Research in Psychology*, 3(2): 77–101.

Brockway, M. and Venturato, L. (2016) 'Breastfeeding beyond infancy: a concept analysis', *Journal of Advanced Nursing*, 72(9): 2003–15.

Bruce, A., Shields, L., Molzahn, A., Beuthin, R., Schick-Makaroff, K. and Shermak, S. (2014) 'Stories of liminality: living with life-threatening illness', *Journal of Holistic Nursing*, 32(1): 35–43.

Buckley, K. M. (2001) 'Long-term breastfeeding: nourishment or nurturance?', *Journal of Human Lactation*, 17(4): 301–12.

Czarniawska, B. and Mazza, C. (2003) 'Consulting as a liminal space', *Human Relations*, 56(3): 267–90.

Douglas, M. (2002 [1966]) *Purity and Danger*, London/New York: Routledge.

Dowling, S. (2009) 'Inside information: researching long-term breastfeeding', *The Practising Midwife*, 12(11): 22–6.

Dowling, S. (2011) 'Online asynchronous and face-to-face interviewing: comparing methods for exploring women's experiences of breastfeeding long-term', in J. Salmons (ed) *Cases in online interview research*, Thousand Oaks, CA/London/New Delhi: Sage, pp 277–96.

Dowling, S. and Brown, A. (2013) 'An exploration of the experiences of mothers who breastfeed long-term: what are the issues and why does it matter?', *Breastfeeding Medicine*, 8 (1): 45–52.

Dowling, S. and Pontin, D. (2017) 'Using liminality to understand mothers' experiences of long-term breastfeeding: "betwixt and between", and "matter out of place"', *Health*, 21(1): 57–75.

Dykes, F. (2009) '"Feeding all the time": women's temporal dilemmas around breastfeeding in hospital', in C. McCourt (ed), *Childbirth, midwifery and concepts of time*, New York/Oxford: Berghahn Books, pp 203–22.

Faircloth, C. (2010a) '"If they want to risk the health and well-being of their child, that's up to them": long-term breastfeeding, risk and maternal identity', *Health, Risk and Society*, 12(4): 357–67.

Faircloth, C. (2010b) '"What science says is best": parenting practices, scientific authority and maternal identity', *Sociological Research Online*, 15(4), www.socresonline.org.uk/15/4/4.html

Faircloth, C. (2011) '"It feels right in my heart": affective accountability in narratives of attachment', *The Sociological Review*, 59(2): 209–91.

Forss, A., Tishelman, C., Widmark, C. and Sachs, L. (2004) 'Women's experience of cervical cancer changes: an unintentional transition from health to liminality', *Sociology of Health and Illness*, 26(3): 306–25.

Granek, L. and Fergus, K. (2012) 'Resistance, agency, and liminality in women's accounts of symptom appraisal and help-seeking upon discovery of a breast irregularity', *Social Science and Medicine*, 75: 1753–61.

Gribble, K. D. (2007) '"As good as chocolate" and "better than ice-cream": how toddler, and older, breastfeeders experience breastfeeding', *Early Child Development and Care*, 179(8): 1067–82.

Gribble, K. D. (2008) 'Long-term breastfeeding: changing attitudes and overcoming challenges', *Breastfeeding Review*, 16(1): 5–15.

Groleau, D., Soulière, M. and Kirmayer, L. J. (2006) 'Breastfeeding and the cultural configuration of social space among Vietnamese immigrant women', *Health and Place*, 12(4): 516–26.

Hills-Bonczyk, S. G., Tromiczak, K. R., Avery, M. D., Potter, S., Savik, K. and Duckett, L. J. (1994) 'Women's experiences with breast-feeding longer than 12 months', *Birth*, 21(4): 206–12.

Horta, B. L. and Victora, C. G. (2013) *Long-term effects of breastfeeding: A systematic review*, Geneva: WHO.

Jordan, J., Price, J. and Prior, L. (2015) 'Disorder and disconnection: parent experiences of liminality when caring for their dying child', *Sociology of Health and Illness*, 37(6): 839–55.

Labbok, M. H. (2012) 'Breastfeeding in public health: what is needed for policy and program action?' in P. H. Smith, B. L. Hausman and M. Labbok (eds) *Beyond health, beyond choice: Breastfeeding constraints and realities*, New Brunswick, NJ: Rutgers University Press, pp 36–50.

Madge, C. and O'Connor, H. (2005) 'Mothers in the making? Exploring liminality in cyber/space', *Transactions of the Institute of British Geographers*, 30(1): 83–97.

Mahon-Daly, P. and Andrews, G. (2002) 'Liminality and breastfeeding: women negotiating space and two bodies', *Health and Place*, 8: 61–76.

McAndrew, F., Thompson, J., Fellows, L., Large, A., Speed, M. and Renfrew, M. J. (2012) 'Infant feeding survey: 2010', NHS Information Centre, http://data.gov.uk/dataset/infant-feeding-survey-2010

McFadden, A., Gavine, A., Renfrew, M. J., Wade, A., Buchanan, P., Taylor, J. L., Veitch, E., Rennie, A. M., Crowther, S. A., Neiman, S. and MacGillivray, S. (2017) 'Support for healthy breastfeeding mothers with healthy term babies', *Cochrane Database of Systematic Reviews*, 2: CD001141.

Morse, J. M. and Harrison, M. J. (1987) 'Social coercion for weaning', *Journal of Nurse-Midwifery*, 32(4): 205–10.

Reamer, S. B. and Sugarman, M. (1987) 'Breast feeding beyond six months: mothers' perceptions of the positive and negative consequences', *Journal of Tropical Pediatrics*, 33: 93–7.

Rempel, L. A. (2004) 'Factors influencing the breastfeeding decisions of long-term breastfeeders', *Journal of Human Lactation*, 20(3): 306–18.

Rollins, N. C., Bhandari, N., Hajeebhoy, N., Horton, S., Lutter, C. K, Martines, J. C., Piwoz, E. G., Richter, L. M. and Victora, C. G., on behalf of The Lancet breastfeeding series group (2016) 'Why invest, and what it will take to improve breastfeeding practices?', *Lancet*, 387(10017): 491–504.

Ryan, K., Todres, L. and Alexander, J. (2011) 'Calling, permission, and fulfillment: the interembodied experience of breastfeeding', *Qualitative Health Research*, 21(6): 731–42.

Sachs, M., Dykes, F. and Carter, B. (2006) 'Feeding by numbers: an ethnographic study of how breastfeeding women understand their babies' weight charts', *International Breastfeeding Journal*, 1(29).

Sears, W. and Sears, M. (2001) *The attachment parenting book*, New York: Little, Brown and Company.

Shattnawi, K. K. (2015) 'Suspended liminality: breastfeeding and becoming a mother in two NICUs', *International Journal of Advanced Nursing Studies*, 4(2): 75–84.

Smale, M. (2001) 'The stigmatisation of breastfeeding', in T. Mason, C. Carlisle, C. Watkins and E. Whitehead (eds) *Stigma and social exclusion in healthcare*, London/New York: Routledge, pp 234–45.

Stearns, C. A. (1999) 'Breastfeeding and the good maternal body', *Gender and Society*, 13(3): 308–25.

Stearns, C. A. (2011) 'Cautionary tales about extended breastfeeding and weaning', *Health Care for Women International*, 32(6): 538–54.

Tomori, C., Palmquist, A. and Dowling, S. (2016) 'Contested moral landscapes: negotiating breastfeeding stigma in breastmilk sharing, nighttime breastfeeding, and long-term breastfeeding in the US and the UK', *Social Science and Medicine*, 168: 178–85.

Trusson, D., Pilnick, A. and Roy, S. (2016) 'A new normal?: women's experiences of biographical disruption and liminality following treatment for early stage breast cancer', *Social Science and Medicine*, 151: 121–9.

Turner, V. (2009 [1969]) *The ritual process: Structure and antistructure*, New York/London: Aldine Transaction.

Unicef UK (2016) 'Protecting health and saving lives: A call to action', https://www.unicef.org.uk/babyfriendly/baby-friendly-resources/advocacy/call-to-action

Van Gennep, A. (1960 [1909]) *The rites of passage*, Chicago, IL: University of Chicago Press.

Victora, C. G., Bahl, R., Barros, A.J.D., França, G.V.A., Horton, S., Krasevec, J., Murch, S., Sankar, M. J., Walker, N., and Rollins, N. C. for the Lancet breastfeeding series group (2016) 'Breastfeeding in the 21st century: epidemiology, mechanisms, and lifelong effect', *Lancet*, 387(10017): 475–90.

FOUR

Weaving breastfeeding practices into policy

Lucila Newell

Introduction

Breastfeeding faces a public health crisis due to the wide gap between policy recommendations and its uptake by women as a practice. At its core, the breastfeeding crisis is a crisis of support that comes at a time when budgetary cuts are deeply affecting breastfeeding support services. I argue here that, if we are to tackle this gap, we need an approach that can incorporate the disparate elements at play in this crisis, an approach that moves away from focusing on breastfeeding solely as a woman's individual behaviour. I propose we focus on the *practice* of breastfeeding.

A practice-based approach moves away from the notion that how people behave is an issue of individual choice (Shove et al, 2012). There is already a diverse array of research that focuses on the health-related and the wider emotional, social and cultural issues that affect breastfeeding, but it tends to be fragmented. What these studies highlight in different ways, is that breastfeeding cannot be properly understood as an issue solely between mothers and babies, but needs to be considered in the web of relations in which diverse mothers and babies are entangled (Newell, 2013). I suggest focusing on practices that can bring together this wealth of research in a way that can inform policy practices.

This chapter explores breastfeeding as a practice through a sociological and geographical perspective. More particularly, I will follow closely Shove's work on social practices (Shove et al, 2012; Shove, 2014) to think about the everyday *practice* of breastfeeding. The aim is to change the type of questions asked about breastfeeding, and to change how the issue is framed, to inspire people to develop alternative policy proposals (Shove et al, 2012). I describe first what a practice-based approach means and looks like, and how it differs from behaviouralist approaches. I then analyse the elements and histories that make up breastfeeding practice today, while outlining its competing practice (feeding using infant formula) and end with thoughts on how these may move policy forward.

Understanding breastfeeding as a practice

Because it is easier to know and recognise a practice than it is to describe and confine it, I use Shove's definition of practices, which characterises them as 'recognisable entities that exist across time and space, that depend on inherently provisional integrations of elements, and that are enacted by cohorts of more and less consistent or faithful carriers' (Shove, 2014: 418). Practices involve the active integration of 'elements'. These include materials, objects and infrastructures, and forms of competence and know-how, images and meanings (Shove, 2014). The task then becomes 'identify[ing] the elements of which such practices are made, their histories, their modes of recruitment and defection' (Shove, 2014: 419). This can be understood with an example from Shove's work. She examines the practice of showering to understand how people might change towards less energy intensive practices, and how showering has changed from being a new practice to an everyday one. She understands showering as an:

> emergent, historically specific outcome of the interweaving of running hot water, bathrooms, concepts of freshness and invigoration, and taken-for-granted skills of personal care (Hand et al, 2005). It is the repeated integration of these elements that makes showering such a regular and normal pursuit for so many people today. (Shove, 2014: 419–20)

Breastfeeding may be understood as a practice of feeding as it fits well with this definition. It is recognisable across space and time, and is/has been enacted by its carriers (women) more or less faithfully over time and space. Elements (materials, objects and infrastructures, forms of competence and know-how, and images and meanings) are different and find different configurations across space and time. I address this in the next section.

A practice-based approach moves away from the notion that how people behave is only a matter of individual choice (Shove et al, 2012). The attitude, behaviour and change components of behavioural change and behaviouralist economic approaches are a common basis for policy making and have an individualistic understanding of action and change

(Barnett, 2010; Shove et al, 2012). These approaches examine how they can persuade people of the importance of an issue at stake. They motivate them to commit to the issue, with its associated values, and remove barriers for that to become the basis of action (Shove et al, 2012). Individuals may be influenced by their context, which becomes a driver or obstacle for action, but this is external to the person. The behavioural change/behaviouralist economic approach does not attend to how the process of doing the practice itself shapes the meanings, and how know-how is formed through this process (Shove et al, 2012). A practice-based approach challenges this notion. It focuses on a number of ideas – how the basis of action is shared, how the process of change is emergent instead of causal, that policy is not external but embedded in the systems of practice it tries to influence – and notices how transferable lessons are limited by specific historical and cultural conditions (Shove et al, 2012). The central focus of intervention ceases to be individual attitudes and action, and shifts to social practices (Shove, 2014).

This does not mean that policy action is irrelevant or incapable of producing change. It places its interventions and its intended/unintended effects in the midst of the ongoing dynamics of practice. Policy at its best may increase the chances of some preferred practices to persist and thrive (Shove et al, 2012). This approach asks: 'How are people drawn into certain practices rather than others, and how do their lives and careers sustain the lives and careers of the practices they reproduce?' (Shove, 2014: 419). This approach addresses systemic challenges to foster long-term changes in what counts as normal and acceptable. When taking a practice-based approach, the target of policy turns to the range of 'elements' of practice, the ways in which practices relate to one another, and the patterns of recruitment and defection (Shove et al, 2012).

With breastfeeding, the emphasis on the drivers and obstacles to individual change may be seen in the emphasis on giving women information about the health benefits of breastfeeding ('breast is best') so that they decide breastfeeding is a better choice. It acts to remove the barriers to changes in women's behaviour, for example, changing discrimination laws and maternity leave entitlements. There are many ways in which policies work on the elements of practice beyond information-giving, for instance, changes to hospital practices and training through the Baby Friendly Initiative, especially its recent relational approach (see 'UK policy context'). These are important, as they alter some of the elements of practice. The practice of giving people information is commendable because it acknowledges individuals as ethical beings who are capable of conscious reflection of values, means and ends (Barnett, 2010). However, it leaves aside the different practice-based ways that people make decisions and decide ethically, that is, the 'habitual form of embodied disposition towards emerging situations' (Barnett, 2010: 1885). Hausman's critique of current advocacy programmes points to this when she argues that 'the advocacy insistence on health information and persuasion as the primary rhetorical emphasis does little to address the difficulties of accommodating breastfeeding as a practice into the busy lives of mothers today' (Hausman, 2004: 280). Some of these missing elements are analysed in the rest of this chapter.

Elements of breastfeeding practice

The first step to understand breastfeeding as a practice is to see which elements are at play, identify the histories of breastfeeding, and explore how these relate to each other in a particular place. I describe here some of the elements present in industrialised societies, including the UK. I then outline how breastfeeding relates to its competing practice: feeding babies with infant formula. Threaded through this analysis are ways in which these practices reproduce each other, and their patterns of recruitment and defection.

The elements of practice are materials, objects and infrastructures, forms of competence and know-how, images and meanings. To understand breastfeeding as an embodied practice, we need to pay attention to women's embodied experience of breastfeeding (Hausman, 2004). Successful breastfeeding partly depends on 'how well the body adapts to physical and psychological exigencies of the practice itself' (Hausman, 2004: 280). And many issues arise through the practice, from problems latching on, mastitis or thrush, to the clash of expectations and reality, especially in its early days (McAndrew et al, 2012; Brown, 2016). Emotions involved in breastfeeding range from joy to pain, shame to pride; these are aroused-in-relation, and from what happens in the practice itself (see Chapters One and Two). Temporal and spatial aspects are crucial parts of breastfeeding practice. Breastfeeding requires mothers and their children to be in close proximity to one another, though this has changed with the advent of breast pumps, bottles, fridges and freezers (Boyer, 2009). And it takes time. It has an irregular regularity throughout day and night; it is practised at a point in time and may require much of the time to be spent being still. Hausman calls it a:

temporal pacing through a 24-hour period, regularity as well as disruption (as in sleep), the calibration of one's own body to the needs of another, frustration due to a blocked or delayed relation, and subjection of one's own felt needs to the perceived needs or demands of another. (Hausman, 2004: 279–80)

This requires perseverance because it is not easily accommodated with current industrialised ways of living (Hausman, 2004; Bartlett, 2005).

Breastfeeding as a practice involves other relations, materials and meanings apart from mothers and babies. It includes women's bodies, infants'/children's bodies, breasts, breast milk, jaw muscles, hormones, breast pads, bras, stretchy and strategic clothes, cover-ups, shawls, muslins, breast pumps, bottles and sterilisers, fridges and freezers, calorie charts, administrative forms in hospitals and those used by midwives and health workers, and so on (Newell, 2013). As the images and meanings associated with breastfeeding have changed, so have the links between these meanings. The nurturing/comfort meaning of breastfeeding remains powerful. It links to parental ideologies and what constitutes a 'good mother'. This comes into conflict with what a 'good' woman does (see Thomson et al, 2015). In the UK, it is also seen as something that more privileged women do, a middle-class practice, or a 'hippie' practice in some areas, and this relates to infrastructures such as maternity leave entitlements, parental ideologies and work structures (see, for instance, Pain et al, 2001; Tomori, 2014; Brown, 2016). Images of breastfeeding have changed over time and space, although some iconic images remain, such as the sacred dyad of Madonna and child. Part of the conflict arises as breasts have become sexualised (Bartlett, 2005; Dowling et al, 2012; Hurst, 2012; Boyer, 2018). This affects how comfortable women are about breastfeeding in public, as the controversies around breastfeeding show. There is a taboo attached to breast milk due the perception of human bodily fluids as being matter out of place in public (Dowling and Pontin, 2017).

The infrastructures linked to breastfeeding practice range from healthcare practices to maternity policies and work structures, shapes of family units, design of urban/rural domestic/public spaces, laws, and to the underlying environment that shapes the practice. Spaces are important when feeding, as different spaces make breastfeeding an issue in particular ways. They help shape the images and meanings of breastfeeding through the media, public debates, campaigns and controversies, discussion in parliament, on forums, social media, blogs, parenting books, public protests, breastfeeding sit-ins, and online activism and protests (Bartlett, 2005; Boyer, 2011; Duckett, 2012; Brown, 2016; Giles 2016; see also Chapter Ten). Not forgetting marketing offices and supermarket shelves, World Health Organization meetings, and policy-making offices. The way breastfeeding is constructed in these spaces plays an important role in shaping these practices.

Competence and know-how about breastfeeding has changed and varied across space and time as breastfeeding has become medicalised. This has changed it from a practice learnt through seeing, modelling and bodily experience, to a professionalised practice mediated by the medical establishment (Bartlett, 2005; Dykes, 2006; Colson, 2010). These elements interrelate with knowledge of care of self, and understandings of how women's bodies work that are centred more on medical information and less on personal bodily and communal experiences (Martin, 2001; Bartlett, 2005). Related to this is the issue of the creation of maternal identities, which shapes how mothers view and construct themselves as breastfeeding mothers (Longhurst, 2008; Faircloth, 2010; Dowling and Pontin, 2017).

These elements are enacted differently in particular places. To really understand how this practice works, we need to investigate how these different elements relate to each other in particular places. Each place and space has its protocol of 'propriety', which intersects with relations that construct particular feeding cultures. For example, breastfeeding in public in the UK is an issue for many mothers. The last Infant Feeding Survey in the UK showed that 45% of mothers felt uncomfortable feeding in front of others, and most acutely in public spaces (McAndrew et al, 2012). Boyer notes how anxiety-provoking public breastfeeding can be for mothers, and how they may feel uncomfortable owing to concerns about embarrassing others (Boyer, 2012, 2018). The anticipation of a negative reception makes mothers anxious. Boyer suggests that these emotional resonances are a barrier for increasing breastfeeding duration rates (Boyer, 2018). Women struggling to breastfeed see bottle feeding with infant formula as a way to avoid the difficulties of public breastfeeding (Boyer, 2018). The fact that many public spaces 'provide little or no provision for the ordinary fulfilment of breastfeeding practices suggests how breastfeeding is excluded from public life, as well as how maternal practices are shaped by public spaces' (Hausman, 2004: 279).

Access to/participation in breastfeeding practice is uneven and shaped by geography, class, ethnicity and mother's age (McAndrew et al, 2012). Questions about why breastfeeding practice is so unevenly carried are relevant here. Following Bourdieu, the chance of becoming a carrier of any practice is intimately linked to 'the social and symbolic significance of participation, and to the highly structured and vastly different opportunities to accumulate and amass the different types of capital required for, and typically generated by participation' (Shove et al, 2012: 65). In the UK and US, there is a difference in who becomes a carrier. Generally, older, more educated women who have a higher socioeconomic status are more likely to breastfeed, though this is different within certain ethnic communities. Boyer (2018) and Groleau, Sigouin and D'Souza (2013) show how for some women breasts constitute sexual capital that helps maintain their identity and power. They are less likely to take breastfeeding up as a practice if they feel it might jeopardise this identity and power. Women who have less of other types of capital (symbolic, cultural, economic) may be more reliant on their partners for financial, social, emotional and housing support (Boyer, 2018). Breastfeeding practice is not attracting women because participation is highly structured in terms of support, and the social and cultural significance of participating is less important for some women compared to what other practices have to offer.

Breastfeeding as a practice loses many of its carriers because deeper issues are not addressed. The numbers of mothers initiating breastfeeding are increasing, but they quickly fall, earlier than women would like (McAndrew et al, 2012). To understand the bigger picture, we also need to see how this practice relates to its contending practice: feeding with infant formula. We should examine this form of feeding babies and its elements to understand how it has secured more women, and to identify the patterns of recruitment and defection to bring more clarity.

Infant formula feeding as competing practice

Formula feeding has not been studied as a practice in so much depth, though the marketing of formula has been shown to be detrimental to breastfeeding (Van Esterik, 1989; Palmer, 2009; Rollins et al, 2016). There is scope to be more curious about formula feeding as a practice. I propose here an approach to study this practice and an outline of some of its elements, but it requires further research and development.

Many studies that pay attention to the practice of formula feeding frame it in a negative way. To move away from this type of analysis, I introduce here Hawkings' (2009) work on plastic bottles. She states that:

> Current political and moral framings of bottled water situate
> it as always already bad. As a relatively new commodity it is

seen to manifest all that is wrong with global corporations and their ruthless exploitation of natural resources and gullible consumers. The problem is, however, that in seeking to politicise the bottle, these approaches deny its constitutive role in social and political life. Instead, they present an array of facts about bottles that establish their status as a problem, and then suggest a range of human or technological interventions aimed at eradicating or controlling them ... The bottled water consumer is implicitly framed as stupid, easily scared by tap water risks and easily seduced by the fantasy of 'organic' water. There is little attempt to explain how a consumer for bottled water is made up or how the bottle, itself, might be involved in framing its markets. The bottle is so over coded as an environmental catastrophe that such modest questions seem almost obscene.' (Hawkings, 2009: 184–5)

There are parallels between what Hawkings says about plastic bottles and feeding babies with infant formula. Analysing mothers who bottle-feed with infant formula from a political economy approach (Palmer, 2009) is a useful activity to mobilise politically and generate changes. It is less good at opening up the repertoire of feelings of everyday practices that make feeding babies with infant formula gain women, allowing for different kinds of politics, and opening up different ways of generating change. Analyses such as Palmer's tend to forget the power of objects and their enrolled meanings in the making of everyday practices.

Political and moral approaches to feeding babies with infant formula are situated as always already bad. It serves to show what is wrong with capitalism, corporations and patriarchy because they undermine women's bodies. It makes women look like victims, gullible and/or pleasing. This is not helping women; it creates divisions, brings guilt, shame and anger, a sense of failure, and defiance in women who adopt feeding with infant formula as a practice (Thomson et al, 2015). If our aim is to support women, these political and moral approaches are failing. We are also failing to understand why the practice of feeding with infant formula has gained more women than breastfeeding, as it does not go deep into what makes the assemblages that make this practice more dominant than breastfeeding.

The materials, objects and infrastructures, forms of competence and know-how, images and meanings that configure the elements of feeding with infant formula as a practice differ from those of breastfeeding. Feeding babies infant formula involves other bodies, because it allows fathers (and other carers) to feed babies. Babies, bottles, teats, dried infant formula powder, packaging, sterilising equipment, hot water and equipment bags are some of the materials and objects involved (Newell, 2013). The practice of feeding with infant formula requires babies' bodies to adapt to this practice. Sometimes this means searching for different brands of infant formula, even though they all must conform to required standards. It requires an initial adjustment to not breastfeeding, but less understanding and adaptation from mothers' bodies in the long-term, although there are new bodily postures and ways of holding bottles that lead to better performance. Feeding infant formula to babies requires a carer to be nearby, but removes the need for mothers to be in close proximity to babies (Boyer, 2009). It is also a practice that takes time, needs regular attendance and works on a 24-hour basis. Its infrastructures link to ways we meet some of our needs in industrialised societies. It creates and relies on retail stores and distribution networks, industrial dairy farming practices, manufacturers and laboratories (see also Chapter Twelve). It creates a market through marketing offices, products and practices, television and other media adverts, plastic products, and household technologies (sterilisers, for instance). There are associated energy sources such as gas and electricity, water distribution infrastructures for potable drinking water from taps, and waste disposal infrastructures.

Feeding with infant formula taps into already established forms of competence and know-how, images and meanings (Shove et al, 2012). It taps into our ease of using technologies, such as sterilisers, and our need to control, measure and be productive. It taps into notions of hygiene and self-care by keeping the body under control (Dowling et al, 2012). Spilling infant formula does not contravene the taboo of bodily fluids leaking from women's bodies (Boyer, 2018). Bottles of infant formula in fridges or supermarkets are not offensive (Boyer, 2009).

The images and meanings that feeding with infant formula taps into are powerful notions of what it means to be a modern woman in industrialised societies. It resonates with notions of independence, productivity and achievement. Earning a living, which gives women independence and reduces their vulnerability, in a society where work and life are mostly separate, means finding ways of feeding a baby while women are away. Formula feeding provides one solution. It relates to women's notion of their sexual capital (Groleau et al, 2013). It is related to meanings about the care of women's appearance and what it means to be a good woman: one who does not show her breasts in public, who is in control of her body and not leaking fluids (Thomson et al, 2015). Notions of fairness are tied to this practice. It taps into a sense of fairness about the division of labour where men and other carers can share the load and joy of feeding babies (Boyer, 2018). It chimes with notions of convenience of feeding in public, as it avoids making others uncomfortable (Boyer, 2018); there is no danger of being told to cover up your breasts or to leave a cafe if you feed with infant formula.

If we follow a practice-based approach, we may understand feeding with infant formula as a particular assemblage. Paraphrasing Shove (2014: 419–20), feeding with infant formula may be seen as an emergent, historically specific outcome from the interweaving of concepts of convenience, propriety and productivity, the appearance of plastic as an everyday material, urban and market infrastructures (tap water, waste collection and so on) as well as women's sense of independence. It is the recurrent integration of these elements that makes feeding with infant formula such an ordinary pursuit for so many women today. Policy has not influenced these wider issues affecting breastfeeding as a practice, especially as it relates to its competing practice. In the next section, I explore ways in which policy could engage with and influence these practices.

How can policy influence these practices?

Policy practices are embedded in the processes that it seeks to influence, which have a life of their own (Shove et al, 2012). However, there are ways to influence some of the meanings, materials, objects and infrastructures, the know-how and competences that these practices encompass. First, breastfeeding needs to be prioritised over feeding with infant formula with processes that generate positive feedback. The focus on behavioural change, on information-giving and targeting individual women, has not changed UK breastfeeding rates enough.

To survive, practices need to secure and maintain resources and practitioners willing and able to keep them alive, but processes of defection are as important as those of recruitment (Shove et al, 2012). Many women stop breastfeeding early, and there are many elements that may cause this, including problems within the practice itself, and in bodily accommodation to this practice. Breastfeeding in public is one of the issues given by women for switching to infant formula in the early weeks (Boyer, 2018). We need to create infrastructures that enable and accommodate women's bodies in public spaces. This means creating spaces and making women feel comfortable, so that they don't feel anxious, embarrassed or shamed in front of others. For public breastfeeding to be ubiquitous, there is a need for different infrastructures, meanings and a sense of competence and trust in women's bodies. Deep sociocultural assumptions need to shift, different images must be generated to challenge perceptions of who is allowed to do what in public spaces and how. This is not the responsibility of the breastfeeding mother. Obviously, this is beyond the scope of policy, but there are ways to influence these elements.

This falls within the challenge to configure a different sense of sexual equality. A notion of female independence that imagines women as female men has big costs; one of them is breastfeeding. Women as female men forgets women's bodily experiences and uniqueness, because 'the ability to act as men in the social sphere (that is, to be autonomous individuals without physiologically dependent others) is to impoverish our expectation of what sexual equality should be' (Hausman, 2004: 282).

Policies can erode elements of undesirable practices, and break the links holding them in place (Shove et al, 2012). What would this look like? Looking at the elements of the competing practices, we can focus on changing the elements of feeding with infant formula as a practice. For instance, manufacturers of infant formula try to escape from its materiality and infrastructures: the use of plastic and oil to create bottles, the use of cow's milk, the dairy industry links, the laboratory connection, the creation of markets and consumers, and the waste (see also Chapter Twelve). This is invisible to most consumers. What is the scope to bring this out? Are there ways that infant formula could be made less convenient?

A radical approach would be to make breastfeeding more accessible and valuable for women less likely to breastfeed. What appears normal, sensible and valuable is shaped in the interaction of personal and institutional practices (Shove et al, 2012). If women are vulnerable with fewer types of capital available, and thus are having to lean in to their sexual capital, could their vulnerability be reduced? How can we build different infrastructures, meanings and support networks that go beyond convincing individual women? We could also learn from the success of the practice of feeding with infant formula at gaining more women. Could some of the elements and associations be used to convince more women to be carriers of a breastfeeding practice? These are a few of the questions that arise by framing the issue in a different way.

Conclusion

Breastfeeding has become a public health issue, but the gap between recommendations and policies encouraging breastfeeding and the actual uptake of breastfeeding as a practice is huge. The aim of this chapter has been to reframe the problem and generate different questions, moving away from individual choice to focus on social practices. It suggests a framework focusing on practices to bring in the wealth of research and perspectives on breastfeeding that focus on the wider emotional, social and cultural issues that affect breastfeeding in a way that can inform policy practices.

This practice-based approach changes the questions and issues to be tackled if we want to support women to breastfeed. It suggests that we need to move away from an individualistic notion of action and change. A practice-based approach highlights the cultural and history-laden trajectories of what people do, which in turn are a product of particular associations of meanings, materials and competences, and the relationship between different practices (Shove et al, 2012). Instead of looking at how to change individual behaviour – in this case, trying to influence women to breastfeed – policy makers, then, would be giving attention to how to influence the range of elements of the practices involved, the ways the practices relate to each other, the career and trajectories of the practices and those who carry them, and the way these practices are reproduced (Shove et al, 2012). I have outlined here some of the elements of breastfeeding as a practice and some elements of its competing practice, formula feeding. I have also shown how different questions arise as we change the way we frame the issue. I argue that more attention is needed to understand the practice of formula feeding, and the links between these competing practices in particular places, in order to try to influence these.

Finally, a practice-based methodology attempts to create change through a more holistic approach. If breastfeeding is to become a priority, there needs to be a more concerted effort across different policy areas, not just those focusing on health. A first step would be to examine how breastfeeding is prioritised/undermined in different areas of policy practice, as policy processes are part of the issue at stake. I have outlined here only a few of them: from health practices in hospitals to the design of public spaces, from infrastructures of consumption to those affecting women's vulnerability or to those relating to environmental sustainability, to name just a few. The aim of this approach is to address systemic challenges so as to encourage long-term changes and to normalise and make certain practices more acceptable. In this case, the aim would be to normalise breastfeeding.

References

Barnett, C. (2010) 'The politics of behaviour change', *Environment and Planning A*, 42(8): 1881–6.

Bartlett, A. (2005) *Breastwork: Rethinking breastfeeding*, Sydney: University of South Wales Press.

Boyer, K. (2009) 'Of care and commodities: breast milk and the new politics of mobile biosubstances', *Progress in Human Geography*, 34(1): 5–20.

Boyer, K. (2011) '"The way to break the taboo is to do the taboo thing", Breastfeeding in public and citizen activism in the UK', *Health and Place*, 17: 430–37.

Boyer, K. (2012) 'Affect, corporeality and the limits of belonging: breastfeeding in public in the contemporary UK', *Health and Place*, 18(3): 552–60.

Boyer, K. (2018) 'The emotional resonances of breastfeeding in public: the role of strangers in breastfeeding practice', *Emotion, Space and Society*, 26: 33–40, http://dx.doi.org/10.1016/j.emospa.2016.09.002

Brown, A. (2016) *Breastfeeding uncovered: Who really decides how we feed our babies?*, London: Pinter and Martin.

Colson, S. (2010) *An introduction to biological nurturing*, Amarillo, TX: Hale Publishing.

Dowling, S. and Pontin, D. (2017) 'Using liminality to understand mothers' experiences of long-term breastfeeding: "betwixt and between", and "matter out of place"', *Health*, 21 (1): 57–75.

Dowling, S., Naidoo, J. and Pontin, D. (2012) 'Breastfeeding in public: women's bodies, women's milk', in P. H. Smith, B. L. Hausman and M. Labbok (eds) *Beyond health, beyond choice: Breastfeeding constraints and realities*, New Brunswick, NJ: Rutgers University Press, pp 249–58.

Duckett, N. D. (2012) *Rethinking the importance of social class: how mass market magazines portray infant feeding*, in P. H. Smith, B. L. Hausman and M. Labbok (eds) *Beyond health, beyond choice: Breastfeeding constraints and realities*, New Brunswick, NJ: Rutgers University Press, pp 236–48.

Dykes, F. (2006) *Breastfeeding in hospital: Mothers, midwives and the production line*, London: Routledge.

Faircloth, C. (2010) '"If they want to risk the health and well-being of their child, that's up to them": long-term breastfeeding, risk and maternal identity', *Health, Risk and Society*, 14: 357–67.

Giles, F. (2016) '"Narcissism gone nuts" or "empowering exhibitionism"? Brelfies, popular culture and breastfeeding's burgeoning publics', Conference presentation, Social experiences of breastfeeding: Building bridges between research and policy, ESRC seminar series, 9 June 2016, University of Cardiff, Wales.

Groleau, D., Sigouin, C. and D'Souza, N. D. (2013) 'Power to negotiate spatial barriers to breastfeeding in a western context: When motherhood meets poverty'. *Health and Place*, 24: 250–59.

Hausman, B. (2004) 'The feminist politics of breastfeeding', *Australian Feminist Studies*, 19 (45): 273–85.

Hawkings, G. (2009) 'The politics of bottled water', *Journal of Cultural Economy*, 2(1): 183–95.

Hurst, C. G. (2012) Sexual or maternal breasts? A feminist view of the contested right to breastfeed publicly, in P. H. Smith, B. L. Hausman and M. Labbok (eds) *Beyond health, beyond choice: Breastfeeding constraints and realities*, New Brunswick, NJ: Rutgers University Press, pp 259–68.

Longhurst, R. (2008) *Maternities: Gender, bodies and spaces*, London: Routledge.

Martin, E. (2001) *The woman in the body: A cultural analysis of reproduction*, Boston, MA: Beacon Press.

McAndrew, F., Thompson, J., Fellows, L., Large, A., Speed, M. and Renfrew, M. J. (2012) 'Infant Feeding Survey 2010', Health and Social Care Information Centre, http://content.digital.nhs.uk/catalogue/PUB08694/Infant-Feeding-Survey-2010-Consolidated-Report.pdf

Newell, L. (2013) 'Disentangling the politics of breastfeeding', *Children's Geographies*, 11 (2): 256–61.

Pain, R., Bailey, C. and Mowl, G. (2001) 'Infant feeding in North East England: contested spaces of reproduction', *Area*, 33: 261–71.

Palmer, G. (2009) *The politics of breastfeeding* (3rd edn), London: Pinter and Martin.

Rollins, N. C., Bhandari, N., Hajeebhoy, N., Horton, S., Lutter, C. K., Martines, J. C., Piwoz, E. G., Richter, L. M. and Victora, C. G. (2016) 'Why invest, and what it will take to improve breastfeeding practices?, *The Lancet*, 387 (10017): 491–504.

Shove, E. (2014) 'Putting practice into policy: reconfiguring questions of consumption and climate change', *Contemporary Social Science*, 9 (4): 415–29.

Shove, E., Sigouin, C. and D'Souza, M. (2012) *The dynamics of social practice: Everyday life and how it changes*, London: Sage.

Smyth, L. (2012) 'The social politics of breastfeeding: norms, situations and policy implications', *Ethics and Social Welfare*, 6 (2): 182–94.

Thomson, G., Ebisch-Burton, K. and Flacking, R. (2015) 'Shame if you do – shame if you don't: women's experiences of infant feeding', *Maternal and Child Nutrition*, 11 (1): 33–46.

Tomori, C. (2014) *Nighttime breastfeeding: An American cultural dilemma*, New York: Berghahn Books.

Van Esterik, J. (1989) *Beyond the breast-bottle controversy*, New Brunswick, NJ: Rutgers University Press.

Breastfeeding and emotions: reflections for policy and practice

Sally Johnson and Sally Tedstone

Introduction

We found a wealth of rich material in these chapters, enough to fuel many conversations and stimulate much reflection. Faced with the constraints of bringing all of this together for one short reflective chapter, we decided to focus on the aspects of the chapters which are the most relevant to the public health outcomes that are the focus of our professional roles, namely, breastfeeding prevalence at six weeks and supporting good perinatal mental health. In particular, we were drawn to the issues of guilt and shame, especially when breastfeeding does not go well, that were discussed by Dawn Leeming and Lisa Smyth (Chapters One and Two). We met to discuss the chapters, and both found that Dawn's insights drawn from the psychological literature helped us make sense of our experience in practice. We've shared some of our conversations below:

Sally T: The distinction Dawn makes between shame and guilt was new to me. I had not given it much consideration before hearing her lecture.

Sally J: This distinction was also new to me. Dawn presents a convincing argument for developing awareness of and sensitivity to those who experience internalised and sometimes intense feelings of shame. However, she balances this with a helpful warning about the dangers of not 'overstating' the 'possibility of shame'. It's important not to overgeneralise, particularly when considering population health.

We were both interested in the ideas Dawn identified from the research on how to help new mothers avoid and resist feeling shame. This became a focus of discussion.

Realistic breastfeeding promotion and education

Sally J: The tide is definitely shifting away from public health campaigns that have 'breast is best' type messages at the centre, but rather promoting services that support women, some of whom may not find it easy to establish breastfeeding. One local campaign, promoting the message of 'go with the flow' was directly inspired by the breastfeeding seminar series. It was intended to challenge the idea of getting your baby into a routine, an idea that in some bestselling books on parenting is synonymous with 'good mothering', and to promote responsive feeding and sensitive, attuned baby-led parenting. This links with Dawn's idea of promoting an 'adjustment period' in breastfeeding – a practical idea that strikes a good balance between acknowledging that there may be difficulties for some while not putting women off because they think it's too difficult. Does that sit comfortably for you in practice?

Sally T: Yes, our focus in maternity services has been to equip staff with the practical skills and knowledge to support breastfeeding effectively. It seems that we need to develop our collective narrative, building on the Unicef Baby Friendly standards and the concept of responsive feeding to widen the discussion to include the adjustment period. There are opportunities here to align with and reinforce information given to parents at the health visitor antenatal contact.

Sally J: This fits in well with work being progressed locally to agree consistent messaging for services supporting families from conception to five years. It's part of a broader agenda to better integrate early years services. The local Public Health team are centrally involved in this work and can help drive change as lead commissioners of health visiting services. We can also discuss the implications at the local Breastfeeding Strategy Group that we both sit on.

Also, where do dads fit in? You'll recall a local project aimed at positively influencing dads' attitudes, beliefs and behaviours in relation to breastfeeding. A theme that came through semi-structured interviews with dads and a subsequent survey highlighted the lack of information available about breastfeeding difficulties and how unprepared they felt. Most dads expressed shocked when their partner experienced breastfeeding problems, never thinking that 'such a natural process' would cause any difficulties. The work culminated in local health visiting and maternity services making changes to how they promote breastfeeding and the development of a resource for dads which acknowledges the challenges of breastfeeding and provides them with ideas for how they can support their partner. The resource has been well received by those dads who are aware of it, but I'm not assured that health professionals are routinely promoting it? What's your observation on the ground?

Sally T: Supporting couples through the transition to parenthood is an important aspect of maternity services, but I fear that where continuity of care is poor this aspect gets lost.

Sally J: Continuity of care is a key area for development identified through the National Maternity Review, so there's potentially a lever for this to change. Local maternity systems (providers, commissioners, public health and service users) are responsible for developing 'Maternity Transformation Plans' in response to several key themes identified through the review.

Dawn also mentions environmental constraints in her chapter. This relates to the local strategic objective of promoting breastfeeding as the cultural norm. This is difficult to penetrate at a local level. The main focus has been increasing the number of venues signed up to the Breastfeeding Welcome scheme. A range of council (local government) run and commissioned venues have signed up, and opportunities are also taken through training to ensure frontline staff have a working understanding of the policy in practice, such as lifeguards in leisure centres. To what extent do you think this makes a difference?

Sally T: It is difficult to measure the impact of this work, but I do feel that as part of a multifaceted approach to supporting breastfeeding, it has its place. Thinking of the conversations you have been having with leisure services about breastfeeding in the pool, potentially many of those staff members were not aware of the importance of breastfeeding for the health of mothers and babies, how often babies feed, and the cultural barriers that women can face. All these small conversations I see as the steps on our journey to cultural change.

We talked at this point about how we could introduce the concept of shame and how it differs from guilt to the breastfeeding strategy group. We also contemplated whether actions were being progressed to support mothers to build resilience against shame.

Supporting mothers in becoming resilient

Sally J: Connection, acceptance and validation underpin the breastfeeding peer support scheme locally. However, there are no mixed-feeding groups, and we have to consider how those who are mixed or bottle feeding also connect, feel accepted and validated about their infant feeding practices. Before we explore this further, it would be helpful to hear from you about the extent to which you think the issues of shame articulated by Dawn and Lisa were helpful to consider in practice.

Sally T: In my role as an infant feeding specialist working in maternity services I am frequently supporting women who are experiencing challenging breastfeeding journeys, and difficult, painful emotions are often part of this. Reflecting on the range of emotional responses I perceive in the women I support, the distinction made between guilt (as making a negative judgement that our behaviour has not met a moral standard) and shame (making a negative judgement of our whole self) feels accurate. There are a number of ways in which these insights are proving valuable in clinical practice. First, understanding that shame is often hidden and as a culture we do not have the language to express it clearly; recognising that, as Dawn states, we need to become attuned to the trickier interpersonal dynamics of shame by paying attention and listening carefully to what women say and do. With this heightened awareness I feel as if my 'shame radar' has been turned on and is becoming more sensitive the more I notice and pay attention. Second, learning about the compass of shame and the different ways women may respond to experiencing feelings of shame (attacking themselves, withdrawing, attacking others) has helped me to understand the different ways women can react to difficult experiences . Finally, I have appreciated Dawn's discussion of how we can support women to be more resilient in the face of an experience which triggers shame. Dawn suggests that connection and validation are likely to be important.

Sally J: Have you any ideas about how we can better support mothers to be more resilient against shame?

Sally T: At the Royal United Hospitals NHS Foundation Trust we have been fortunate to be able to work collaboratively with local health visitor colleagues in the development of a specialist service for women with significant breastfeeding challenges. We have gently felt our way with this, wanting to develop a service that does not further medicalise the situation. We aimed to give mothers the time, space and practical support they need, and to link them with other mothers. What has evolved is the Bath Area Early Feeding Circle, a 'by referral' drop-in session where mothers and babies (and the occasional partner) are supported alongside other mothers. It's halfway between a specialist clinic and a peer support group. Early evaluation is showing us that the peer support aspect of this service is immensely valuable. Women report that it is the only place they go where they don't feel like the only one experiencing difficulties. Being with other women who are also struggling feels positive; in Dawn's language, it provides connection and validation.

Sally J: It sounds as though you and those involved in this work are already applying some of the ideas Dawn espouses. You talked earlier about ensuring staff are skilled up to support breastfeeding effectively. There may be another opportunity to link with a theme from the National Maternity Review: better personalised and women-centred care. The skills required to improve care in this way are undoubtedly relevant to adopting the person-centred approach to breastfeeding referred to by Dawn. It's also worth highlighting the potential wider benefits of developing good 'shame antennae' for those working with women from more vulnerable/marginalised groups who may already feel stigmatised and criticised.

Supporting health professionals

Sally J: Dawn also talks about how healthcare professionals or others supporting breastfeeding are not immune to involvement in shame cycles. Do you think this would need to be considered through any training delivered?

Sally T: Absolutely, my instinct is that what we sometime refer to as 'baggage', the unresolved feelings that some health professionals carry around with them in relation to their early mothering and feeding experiences, may contain a significant element of shame. In addition, I suspect that there may be elements of shame created by very pressured work environments. Knowing that the care you are giving is less than the best but feeling powerless to change the situation could be experienced as shameful by some.

How to best support staff experiencing shame in the personal or professional domain is a question I am asking myself. I have not come up with any answers yet, but I do know it won't be simply a couple of PowerPoint slides that's the answer. I am sure there is plenty we have to learn from our colleagues in the voluntary sector on handling these issues with emotional intelligence.

We were both convinced that there was important learning to be drawn from the work on shame and guilt and potentially change in practice, but we were challenged initially by what we could realistically do to progress this, particularly in a climate of financial pressure and limited resource.

Going forward

The second time we met, after time to reflect, the ideas started to materialise. We thought about introducing the concept of shame at a future Breastfeeding Strategy Group meeting and discussing the implications for the work being progressed locally. We both responded positively to the idea of action learning sets as a supportive and useful mechanism to explore the concept of shame, and to help practitioners develop good 'shame antennae'. To help with consistency of approach and to take the opportunity to strengthen maternity–health visiting relationships the sets would be mixed. Action learning sets would provide supportive, safe, confidential, listening environments within which practitioners would share positive and challenging experiences. The environment would model the safe, confidential and supportive environments that women who may be feeling shame need to articulate their emotions.

We acknowledged that shame and how it differs from guilt is a topic that requires careful, considered introduction, preferably by an expert. So, we decided to plan an event and invite key speakers on the subject, including Dawn, to attend. We'd work beforehand to promote the event and the action learning sets would follow.

Finally, we reflected on how positive and productive it has been to work together writing this commentary. The process has given us a focus and structure and the motivation and positivity experienced at each meeting has generated a shared energy that we both believe will propel this work forward. We're clear that our ultimate goal is to improve outcomes for women.

PART II

Cultures of Breastfeeding

'Missing milk': an exploration of migrant mothers' experiences of infant feeding in the UK

Louise Condon

Introduction

In this chapter, the experiences of parents born abroad who are raising a child in the UK are explored. It is recognised that work, paid and unpaid, can pose challenges to exclusive and even partial breastfeeding (Hawkins et al, 2007; Chuang et al, 2010), and such challenges are exacerbated when mothers are migrants and live in precarious social and financial circumstances. A complex mixture of factors influences infant feeding behaviours, including ethnicity, health beliefs and financial demands; and the economic necessity to return to work soon after delivery has been previously identified as a factor reducing migrant women's ability to breastfeed (Schmied et al, 2012). Who migrants are and what is known about their breastfeeding and weaning behaviours will be addressed, and I will then reflect upon two empirical studies conducted with migrant parents in the South West of England. In this way, the voices of migrants from a variety of migrant backgrounds will be heard and their experiences explored in depth. Throughout the chapter the concept of 'missing milk' will be discussed, and the consequences for babies, parents and society raised. 'Missing milk' is the breast milk that babies would customarily have received, which has decreased following migration.

Who are migrants?

The United Nations defines a migrant as a person born abroad and who intends to stay in the country of settlement for at least one year (UNSC, 1998). The vast majority of migrants to the UK come to work (Rutter, 2015). Migrants from European Union (EU) member states have free movement among states, but non-EU migrants are subject to immigration controls (Vargas-Silva and Markaki, 2017). Migrant workers differ from UK-born workers in being younger (over 30% are aged 25–35 years), less likely to be unemployed and more highly educated (Rienzo, 2017). All migrants are more likely to be in employment for which they are overqualified (ONS, 2016a).

In 2015, 13.3% of the usually resident population of the UK were born abroad (ONS, 2016b), which is comparable to France (12%) and Germany (14%), and less than some European countries, for example, Switzerland (29%) (United Nations, 2015). Migration to the UK has been increasing since the 1990s, and the accession of new member states to the EU (Poland in 2004 and Romania in 2007) has led to increased numbers from Eastern Europe. Currently around 30% of UK migrants were born in other EU member states and 20% are from South Asia (India, Pakistan, Bangladesh and Sri Lanka) (Rutter, 2015). In the UK, the number of children born to migrant parents is rapidly increasing, with 27.5% of live births in 2015 being to mothers born outside the UK (ONS, 2016b).

So far, we have been discussing migrants as a homogeneous group, but it is well recognised that there are wide differences between migrants according to their history, background and language (Jayaweera and Quigley, 2010). These differences impact upon key aspects of their post-migration life, such as health, employment and housing. A salient point to recall is that while being foreign-born is a permanent circumstance, citizenship and ethnicity are not static conditions. Some migrants adopt UK citizenship, and ethnicity is not a precise classification, being linked to physical appearance and religious affiliation, but also to subjective identification and stereotyping (Modood et al, 1997). An individual's views on their ethnicity may change over time, or even in different circumstances (Anthias and Yuval-Davis, 1992), which affects self-reporting of ethnicity.

The health of migrants and their children

It is difficult to gain a clear picture of the health of migrants in the UK because much existing evidence on health takes into account ethnic group but not country of birth, length of residence or immigration status (Jayaweera, 2014). While mortality data is recorded according to country of birth, morbidity data in hospital records usually records ethnicity (Jayweera, 2014). Statistics need careful interpretation to ensure they are correctly understood; for instance, an analysis of migrant mothers in the Millennium Cohort Study showed higher rates of those born abroad receiving no antenatal care compared with UK-born mothers. However, regression analysis revealed that the strongest predictors of reporting no antenatal care were being of younger age, lower educational or occupational class and living in a ward where at least 30% of the population were from black and minority ethnic (BME) groups (Jayaweera and Quigley, 2010).

Health outcomes vary according to migration histories and experience, but current evidence suggests poorer health outcomes overall for migrants (Nielsen and Krasnik, 2010; Jayaweera, 2014). The diversity of migrants' backgrounds and experiences (including country of origin, socioeconomic circumstances, legal status and length of residence) has implications for health and needs, and access to healthcare (Jayaweera and Quigley, 2010). The rising number of children of migrants has attracted comment in the popular media as well as in policy discourse of all political colours (Cangiano, 2016; Express, 2016; Migration Watch, 2016). An ONS Bulletin comments on birth rate among migrants:

> The rising percentage of births to women born outside the UK is largely due to foreign born women making up an increasing share of the female population of childbearing age in England and Wales. Part of the reason for this is that migrants are more likely to be working-age adults rather than children or older people. Alongside their increasing share of the population, higher fertility among women born outside the UK has also had an impact. (McLaren in ONS, 2016c: 2)

Many migrants are relatively healthy upon arrival compared with the resident population, but their health status can decline in the receiving society (Rechel et al, 2013). Health issues include maternal and child health, and the health consequences of poor housing and unsafe working conditions in some industries employing migrants (McKay et al, 2006; Perry, 2012). In addition, research suggests that the health behaviours of migrants can deteriorate over time in countries of settlement, particularly in terms of 'lifestyle' choices such as smoking, drinking alcohol and eating a diet high in fat (Hawkins et al, 2008; Delavari et al, 2013; Sanou et al, 2014). This accords with the concept of the 'immigrant paradox' by which immigrants are observed to have healthier behaviours on arrival than subsequently (Sussner et al, 2008).

Relatively little research exists on the health of the children of migrants, as current research and policy are predominantly concerned with ethnic equalities in health (Jayaweera, 2010). Obesity is increasing among migrant populations in high-income countries (Delavari et al, 2013), including childhood obesity (Labree et al, 2011). This systematic review showed that in most of the European countries, migrant children, especially non-Europeans, are at higher risk of being overweight or obese than their native counterparts; the problem of classifying migrant and native children was a limitation. The authors claim that as overweight and obese children are at risk of many chronic health problems, further research is urgently needed in order to develop preventive interventions (Labree et al, 2011).

What is known about infant feeding behaviours in migrant families?

Current infant feeding recommendations are to breastfeed exclusively to six months (WHO, 2003; DH, 2009), then to give home-prepared food such as meat, fish, vegetables and fruit (NICE, 2008), continuing breastfeeding to around one (DH, 2009) or two years of age (WHO, 2003). None of these recommendations is well observed in practice in the UK, with 75% of babies having weaning foods, usually purees or mashed food, by five months and only 1% of mothers breastfeeding exclusively to six months (McAndrew et al, 2012). Infant feeding behaviours impact upon health throughout the lifespan, as breastfed infants have lower risks of morbidity and mortality (Ip et al, 2009; Horta and Victora, 2013), and babies breastfed for at least four months are less likely to be overweight or obese in later childhood (Wallby et al, 2017). Timing and type of solid foods influence both the extent of breastfeeding and diet in later childhood (Northstone et al, 2001; Coulthard et al, 2009). As the World Health Organization points out:

> Lack of breastfeeding – and especially lack of exclusive breastfeeding during the first half-year of life – are important risk factors for infant and childhood morbidity and mortality that are only compounded by inappropriate complementary feeding. (WHO, 2003: v)

Shorter duration of breastfeeding also has an impact upon maternal health. Mothers who breastfeed have a reduced risk of diabetes and some cancers, with greater duration of breastfeeding decreasing risks (Ip et al, 2009; Liu et al, 2010).

Like many surveys, the now discontinued UK Infant Feeding Survey did not distinguish between British-born or migrant participants or provide information about the length of time since migration (Kelly et al, 2006; McAndrew et al, 2012). In the UK, the highest rates of breastfeeding in the white population are found among older mothers in professional employment; however, mothers from minority ethnic groups are more likely to breastfeed irrespective of socioeconomic background (McAndrew et al, 2012). This is remarkable when the strength of the link between socioeconomic circumstances and infant feeding behaviours in the white UK population is considered.

Higher breastfeeding rates among migrant mothers cannot be taken for granted, however. Research suggests that mothers migrating to the UK are more likely to pursue optimal breastfeeding behaviours on arrival than after settlement (Evans et al, 1976), with migrant mothers 5% less likely to breastfeed to four months for every additional five years spent in the UK (Hawkins et al, 2008). Thus, babies are 'missing milk' which they would have benefited from if their mothers had continued with their pre-migration feeding patterns. This adds to the health inequalities experienced by migrants and their children.

Why do infant feeding practices change post migration?

The reason for the decline in breastfeeding post migration in the US and Europe is much debated. Changes in health behaviours may be due to 'acculturation' (adopting the behaviours of the host society), or structural barriers to good health such as low income, poor housing and work, reduced access to healthcare, and cultural insensitivity. Acculturation has been defined as 'changes in one's cultural patterns to those of the host society' (Spector, 2010: 19) and the concept has been used to explain the changing pattern of infant feeding among Hispanic people in the US (Gibson et al, 2005; Sussner et al, 2008; Barcelona de Mendoza et al, 2015). In a large UK survey, mothers from ethnic minority groups who spoke English at home were less likely to breastfeed (Kelly et al, 2006), and Choudhry and Wallace (2012) found that mothers who rarely spoke English and socialised mainly within their own cultural community were little influenced by the UK culture of giving infant formula by bottle. Other qualitative studies suggest that feeding behaviours are subject to change over time as women adopt more Western habits of infant feeding (Condon et al, 2003; Ingram et al, 2008). There is some evidence that fear of racism can contribute to the erosion of breastfeeding. One mother from Pakistan said:

> "They want Asian women to breastfeed, but if you breastfeed in public they might say, 'Look at her, she does it anywhere.'" (Condon et al, 2003: 348)

Critics who oppose the use of culture as a research variable have argued that it promotes an individualistic approach to health, obscuring the effects of social class, stress and social exclusion, all social disadvantages to which ethnic minority groups are very liable (MacLachlan, 2006). Hunt, Schneider and Comer (2004) suggest that researchers who subscribe to the concept of acculturation make presumptions about the supposed cultural characteristics of the group studied, as well as failing to define what constitutes the host or 'mainstream' society. Considering the health behaviours of migrants, Jayaweera and Quigley (2010) conclude that models of acculturation have theoretical and empirical limitations.

What are migrant parents' views on infant feeding post migration?

In this section, I look in detail at two studies to gain a more highly nuanced picture of how infant feeding behaviours are influenced by the context of family life post migration and contribute to a more general understanding of the impact of culture upon infant feeding. This is necessary because a broad-brush approach obscures the profound differences between diverse migrant groups. Both qualitative research projects sought to explore the experiences of migrant parents in feeding their preschool children and their views on the extent to which culture and ethnicity influence infant feeding. All parents interviewed were recent migrants with children either born abroad or in the UK, and both studies included Roma participants, the Roma being uniquely disadvantaged and socially excluded migrants (European Union Agency for Fundamental Rights, 2014).

Study 1: Changing feeding practices among migrant Roma mothers

Roma people have a Gypsy background, with a shared language, cultural practices and history of nomadism (Van Cleemput and Parry, 2001). Numbers of Roma people migrating from continental Europe to the UK have increased since EU expansion in 2004 (ONS, 2016a), and it is estimated that there are now around 200,000 Roma people living in the UK (Brown et al, 2014). Roma people have poorer health than other ethnic groups (Gualdi-Russo et al, 2009; Janevic et al, 2012) and poorer access to healthcare (Colombini et al, 2012). Janevic et al (2010) highlight breastfeeding as a positive health behaviour in the Roma population. For this reason, Roma migrants are of interest when studying infant feeding post migration. In this study (Condon and Salmon, 2015) Roma mothers and grandmothers (n = 22) living in South West England took part in semi-structured interviews focused on breastfeeding and introduction of solid foods. All had migrated from Romania. Data were collected between November 2011 and February 2012.

Views of breastfeeding among Roma participants were highly positive and focused holistically on the general healthiness, ease and convenience of breastfeeding, and the baby's enjoyment:

> 'It is better to breastfeed because it is healthier.' (Roma 2, mother)

> 'Mother's milk is better. We don't give the bottle, you just put the breast in his mouth and that's it, you don't bother with making it.' (Roma 6, mother)

> 'I don't know how to spell it out, it's one of the nicest things a baby can have.' (Roma 11, mother) (Condon, 2015)

Mothers unanimously considered that breastfeeding was healthier than giving infant formula, but did not cite evidence-based benefits of breastfeeding, such as protection from disease for either babies or mothers. Instead, breastfeeding was referred to as a customary feeding method and a community norm: "We raise them with the breast." (Roma 10, grandmother) (Condon and Salmon, 2015: 789).

Mothers described observing breastfeeding as a common part of everyday life, which meant that when they fed their own children they had positive role models. If mothers did experience problems, expertise was at hand:

> 'I saw ... other women how they were doing it, married women, and I observed them and I just knew how to do it.' (Roma 1, mother)

> 'My mum showed him my breasts and she was showing this is how you do it ... Then you take it out and you ... pat him and when you feed him you put him like this.' (Roma 4, mother)

> 'My mother and mother-in-law helped me with my first child until I knew what to do.' (Roma 7, grandmother) (Condon, 2015)

Grandmothers described a tradition of breastfeeding to around two years, with solid foods, such as polenta, pork and nettle soup, introduced at around five to six months. Thus, customary practices described by Roma women conformed to WHO (2003) infant feeding guidelines and were superior to usual infant feeding practices in the UK. However, once in the UK, infant feeding practices could change, often due to work, both paid and unpaid, which took mothers away from breastfeeding responsively. One mother rejoiced that she was not required to sell newspapers on the street, but had the luxury of staying at home to care for her children while her husband worked:

> 'Some bottle-feed their babies and they have other occupations like selling newspapers or doing something to get money ... I just stay at home and take care of the children and my husband goes and works ... I'd rather stay at home.' (Roma 1, mother) (Condon and Salmon, 2015: 791)

The change from breastfeeding to giving infant formula by bottle was described by one grandmother as a part of a process of younger generations becoming more 'civilised': "It has changed. We were giving just breast and now these ones got civilised they give them bottles" (Roma 10, grandmother) (Condon and Salmon, 2015: 791).

Some Roma mothers described mixed feeding from birth once in the UK, with infant formula introduced in the early weeks; often this was done to facilitate work, by allowing another family member to feed the baby. In place of the homemade foods, commercially manufactured baby foods in jars were given as a weaning food, often puddings such as egg custard. For some, the move to solids was as early as four weeks. Mothers who gave both breast milk and infant formula substitutes described problems such as not having enough breast milk, babies displaying nipple confusion and breast aversion, and babies suffering from constipation. When asked the reasons for introducing infant formula substitutes and commercial baby foods, some mothers replied that this was because these were now affordable:

> 'In Romania I didn't have the possibility to buy all the things I needed to bottle-feed, so that's why I breastfed.' (Roma 7, grandmother)

> 'In Romania I did not have enough money for baby food; I had to feed the same food as everyone else.' (Roma 11, mother) (Condon and Salmon, 2015: 791)

Public breastfeeding was avoided by mothers who had lived longer in the UK, and one respondent referred to feeding outside the home as signalling the poverty and disadvantage they aspired to leave behind:

> '[In Romania] the poor ones, the ones that don't have the money to buy powder milk and bottles, then yes they would breastfeed outside the house but the rich ones wouldn't.' (Roma 9, mother) (Condon, 2015)

It is apparent that while there is a cultural tradition of breastfeeding in the Roma community, this is linked inextricably to structural factors such as poverty. Coupled with a desire to follow the social norms of the host country, this contributes to reduced duration of exclusive breastfeeding in the UK.

Study 2: Understanding the context of infant feeding for migrant parents

The second project (Condon and McClean, 2016) differs in that participants were from a variety of migrant groups, from the European Union (Polish, Romanian and Roma) and from more established UK minority communities (Somali and Pakistani). This study aimed to explore how parents keep their preschool children healthy post migration, and five monocultural focus groups were held with parents (n = 28) who had migrated to the UK within the last 10 years. Somali and Pakistani groups consisted solely of mothers, while some fathers attended all European groups. Both Romanian and Romanian Roma participants were included to provide additional context on the migrant experience, as the groups have very different living and working conditions in their country of origin (European Union Agency for Fundamental Rights, 2014).

In this project, a more contextual approach was taken to infant feeding, with exploration of work, housing and leisure pursuits post migration. While wages were higher in the UK, parents found it difficult to find jobs which matched their level of education – "I was finish a Master's degree in administration and in England I am a cleaner" (Polish mother) – and childcare and housing costs were much higher than in their countries of birth. Romanian mothers compared British maternity pay unfavourably with more generous benefits available for mothers in Romania, which influenced how they cared for their child:

'In Romania when you go on maternity you are paid for two years ... you get a month, like a normal wage every month for two years ... it helps a lot. You have time to spend with your child, you have time to see the child grow up, when here maybe in six months you are forced to go back to work.' (Romanian group) (Condon, 2015: np)

Roma mothers, who said they did not receive maternity pay in Romania, again described greater choice of feeding methods once earning more money in the UK:

'In Romania, even if you want to bottle-feed your child you don't have money to buy it, so you have to breastfeed even if you want to or not, but here you do have two options. You can breastfeed, and you can bottle-feed as well because you can afford this; you have more money.' (Roma group) (Condon and McClean, 2016: 459)

None of the Somali or Pakistani participants were working outside of the home, but the shift from living with extended families in their countries of origin influenced their infant feeding practices. Somali mothers described the loss of cultural traditions, such as 40 days' rest after having a baby, which they perceived as leading to an inadequate milk supply:

'Mother when she have baby there, because she was having a lot of rest ... getting support from the family, she was producing much more milk, but here you know, you have a baby two days ago but you have to do all the chores again, taking children to school, walking to the clinic, so you might not produce much milk, so that's why maybe they bottle-feed as well.' (Somali mother 2, age 34) (Condon and McClean, 2016: 459)

Mothers in the Pakistani focus group described breastfeeding as more problematic in the UK because mothers were inhibited from breastfeeding while living in small, shared family houses, compared with houses 'back home' which offered more space for women to feed in private:

'Everybody breastfeeds back home ... a lot of mums want to breastfeed here ... [but] because we are living in a joint family ... they get embarrassed. They can't breastfeed in front of their father-in-law [or] brother-in-law, you know.' (Pakistani mother 4, age 29) (Condon and McClean, 2016: 459)

These findings demonstrate how, within the context of migrants' lives, decisions are made about infant feeding which impact upon the quantity of breast milk babies receive when parents migrate to the UK. Changes in work, social relationships and community structures impact upon the choices parents make about how to feed their babies, and ceasing of traditional cultural practices also plays a part. As has been previously found, migrant women report a clash between their individual beliefs and practices and the dominant practices in the new country, and those who value but do not have access to traditional postpartum practices are more likely to cease breastfeeding (Schmied et al, 2012).

Discussion

It is apparent that babies of migrant mothers are 'missing milk', as duration of breastfeeding is shorter and infant formula substitutes are introduced to allow mothers to work within and outside the home. The example of seeing easy, successful breastfeeding practised routinely by familiar others —the best sort of breastfeeding promotion (Hoddinott and Pill, 1999) – is therefore lost. In addition, solids are given earlier and are of poorer quality; often commercially manufactured sweet baby foods are given in place of savoury homemade foods. Thus, feeding methods which are akin to those of the most advantaged social groups in the UK are being abandoned post migration, in place of inferior feeding practices. Remarkably, parents in both empirical studies appeared unaware of the health consequences of this deterioration in infant feeding for babies and their mothers.

The loss of high-quality feeding practices is lamentable, in view of the disadvantage and social isolation experienced by many migrant parents. Participants in both studies described precarious lives of poorly paid work, coupled with high housing costs and expensive childcare, and there is no reason to think these experiences are atypical of the migrant population (Netto et al, 2011, Pemberton et al, 2014). Structural factors therefore shape the environment in which migrant mothers feed their babies (MacLachlan, 2006). Losing healthy behaviours, which contribute to the short- and long-term health of children and their mothers, adds to health inequalities and the societal burden of ill health. Although obesity is increasing among migrants and their children, particularly those from ethnic minority groups (Renzaho et al, 2008; Labree et al, 2011; Delavari et al, 2013), the extent to which this relates to changes in infant feeding practices is as yet insufficiently explored.

Bhopal (2007) suggests that research into ethnicity and health is of poor quality if it is based upon stereotypes and general impressions, with insufficient consideration of underlying factors such as language, religion and family origins. The studies discussed in this chapter demonstrate an overall declining ability to maintain healthy breastfeeding and weaning behaviours post migration among women from a variety of ethnic and national groups. It highlights the particular needs of Roma people in comparison to other migrants: they experience the worst living and working conditions, yet are losing the protective effects of exclusive breastfeeding for mothers and babies. Despite a tradition of easy and uncontentious breastfeeding, pressure to conform to the dominant bottle-feeding norms leads to changes in behaviours, such as avoiding breastfeeding outside the home. Roma migrants' fragile economic and social status within a society which profoundly discriminates against gypsies (Equality and Human Rights Commission, 2016) increases the desire to avoid activities which are seen as deviant and stigmatising. In contrast with Choudhry and Wallace's (2012) study of infant feeding among South Asian women living in the UK, Roma mothers, while speaking little English and socialising only within their community, appear highly influenced by the UK culture of giving formula by bottle.

As yet there is little focus in local and national strategies on promoting the maintenance of breastfeeding among migrant women, and therefore opportunities to halt the decline may be lost. Unlike the majority population, the challenge in promoting breastfeeding among migrant groups is to support existing practices; however, this does not appear to be an easy task for health professionals. UK studies have shown that maternity services can lack cultural sensitivity, with health professionals viewing ethnic minorities as stereotypical homogeneous groups (McFadden et al, 2012). Abbott and Riga (2007) additionally found insufficient appreciation of the effects of poverty upon lifestyle and access to health services. The challenge for health professionals offering health promotion is to maintain healthy behaviours while respecting the cultural beliefs which lie behind these behaviours, and recognising the difficulties migrants often experience in their daily lives at home and work.

Conclusion

We who promote breastfeeding in the UK can fail to overcome the linguistic, cultural and socioeconomic barriers which prevent migrant mothers receiving the same level of breastfeeding education and promotion as others. Many barriers to optimal infant feeding among migrants differ from those of the majority population, so more innovative and targeted techniques are needed to address issues which are specific to individual migrant communities, such as the nature of women's work. Universal healthy child programmes offer an opportunity for health professionals to provide culturally informed and responsive services to migrant families in order to promote optimal infant feeding.

References

Abbott, S. and Riga, M. (2007) 'Delivering services to the Bangladeshi community: the views of healthcare professionals in East London', *Public Health*, 121 (12): 935–41.

Anthias, F. and Yuval-Davis, N. (1992) *Racialized boundaries: Race, nation, gender, colour and class and the anti-racist struggle*, London: Routledge.

Barcelona de Mendoza, V., Harville, E., Theall, K., Buekens, P. and Chasan-Taber, L. (2015) 'Acculturation and intention to breastfeed among a population of predominantly Puerto Rican women', *Birth*, 43 (1): 78–85.

Bhopal, R. (2007) *Ethnicity, race and health in multicultural societies*, Oxford: Oxford University Press.

Brown, P., Martin, P. and Scullion, L. (2014) 'Migrant Roma in the United Kingdom and the need to estimate population size', *People, Place and Policy Online*, 8 (1): 19–33.

Cangiano, A. (2016) 'The impact of migration on UK population growth', The Migration Observatory, www.migrationobservatory. ox.ac.uk/resources/briefings/the-impact-of-migration-on-uk-population-growth

Choudhry, K. and Wallace, L. (2012) '"Breast is not always best": South Asian women's experiences of infant feeding in the UK within an acculturation framework', *Maternal and Child Nutrition*, 8: 72–87.

Chuang, C., Chang, P. and Chen, Y. (2010) 'Maternal return to work and breastfeeding: a population-based cohort study', *International Journal of Nursing Studies*, 4: 461–74.

Colombini, M., Rechel, B. and Mayhew, S. (2012) 'Access of Roma to sexual and reproductive health services: qualitative findings from Albania, Bulgaria and Macedonia', *Global Public Health*, 7: 522–34.

Condon, L. (2015) '"Missing milk": an exploration of migrant mothers' experiences of breastfeeding in England', Conference presentation, Breastfeeding, wage-work and social exclusion, ESRC seminar series, 4 November 2015, Bristol.

Condon, L. and McClean, S. (2016) 'Maintaining pre-school children's health and wellbeing in the UK: a qualitative study of the views of migrant parents', *Journal of Public Health*, 39(3): 455–63.

Condon, L. and Salmon, D. (2015) 'You likes your way, we got our own way: gypsies and Travellers' views on infant feeding and health professional support', *Health Expectations*, 18 (5): 784–95.

Condon, L., Ingram, J., Hamid, N. and Hussein, A. (2003) 'Cultural influences on breastfeeding and weaning', *Community Practitioner*, 76: 344–9.

Coulthard, H., Harris, G. and Emmett, P. (2009) 'Delayed introduction of lumpy foods to children during the complementary feeding period affects child's food acceptance and feeding at seven years of age', *Maternal and Child Nutrition*, 5: 75–85.

Delavari, M., Sonderlund, A., Swinburn, B., Mellor, D. and Renzaho, A. (2013) 'Acculturation and obesity among migrant populations in high income countries: a systematic review', *BMC Public Health*, 13: 458.

Department of Health (2009) *Healthy Child Programme: Pregnancy and the first five years of life*, London: Department of Health.

Equality and Human Rights Commission (2016) 'England's most disadvantaged groups: Gypsies, Travellers and Roma', https://www.equalityhumanrights.com/sites/default/files/ief_gypsies_travellers_and_roma.pdf

European Union Agency for Fundamental Rights (2014) 'Poverty and employment: the situation of Roma in 11 EU member states', Luxembourg: European Union Agency for Fundamental Rights.

Evans, N., Walpole, I. R., Qureshi, M. U., Memon, M. H. and Everly Jones, H. (1976) 'Lack of breast feeding and early weaning in infants of Asian immigrants to Wolverhampton', *Archives of Disease in Childhood*, 51 (8): 608–12.

Express (2016) 'Number of migrant babies born in the UK soar to new record high', www.express.co.uk/news/uk/606926/Number-migrant-babies-born-UK-SOAR-new-record-high

Gibson, M., Diaz V., Mainous, A. and Geesey, M. (2005) 'Prevalence of breastfeeding and acculturation in Hispanics: results from the NHANES 1999–2000 study', *Birth*, 32: 93–98.

Gualdi-Russo, E., Zironi, A., Dallari, G. and Toselli, S. (2009) 'Migration and health in Italy: a multiethnic adult sample', *Journal of Travel Medicine*, 16: 88–95.

Hawkins, S., Griffiths, L., Dezateux, C. and Law, C. (2007) 'The impact of maternal employment on breast-feeding duration in the UK Millennium Cohort Study', *Public Health Nutrition*, 10 (9): 891–6.

Hawkins, S., Lamb, K., Cole, T. and Law, C. (2008) 'Influence of moving to the UK on maternal health behaviours: prospective cohort study', *British Medical Journal*, 336(7652): 1052.

Hoddinott, P. and Pill, R. (1999) 'Qualitative study of decisions about infant feeding among women in east end of London', *British Medical Journal*, 318(7175): 30–34.

Horta, B. and Victora, C. (2013) 'Long-term effects of breastfeeding: a systematic review', http://biblio.szoptatasert.hu/sites/default/files/Long-term_effects_of_breastfeeding_WHO2013.pdf

Hunt, L., Schneider, S. and Comer, B. (2004) 'Should "acculturation" be a variable in health research? A critical review of research on US Hispanics', *Social Science and Medicine*, 59 (5): 973–86.

Ingram, J., Cann, K., Peacock, J. and Potter, B. (2008) 'Exploring the barriers to exclusive breastfeeding in black and minority ethnic groups and young mothers in the UK', *Maternal and Child Nutrition*, 4: 171–80.

Ip, S., Chung, M., Raman, G., Trikalinos, T. A. and Lau, J. (2009) 'A summary of the Agency for Healthcare Research and Quality's evidence report on breastfeeding in developed countries', *Breastfeeding Medicine*, 4 (S1): S–17.

Janevic, T., Petrovic, O., Bjelic, I. and Kubera, A. (2010) 'Risk factors for childhood malnutrition in Roma settlements in Serbia', *BMC Public Health*, 10: 509.

Janevic, T., Jankovic, J. and Bradley, E. (2012) 'Socioeconomic position, gender, and inequalities in self-rated health between Roma and non-Roma in Serbia', *International Journal of Public Health*, 57: 49–55.

Jayaweera, H. (2010) *Health and access to health care of migrants in the UK*, London: Race Equality Foundation.

Jayaweera, H. (2014) 'Health of migrants in the UK: What do we know?', The Migration Observatory, www.migrationobservatory.ox.ac.uk/resources/briefings/health-of-migrants-in-the-uk-what-do-we-know

Jayaweera, H. and Quigley, M. (2010) 'Health status, health behaviour and healthcare use among migrants in the UK: evidence from mothers in the Millennium Cohort Study', *Social Science and Medicine*, 71: 1002–10.

Kelly, Y., Watt, R. and Nazroo, J. (2006) 'Racial/ethnic differences in breastfeeding initiation and continuation in the United Kingdom and comparison with findings in the United States', *Pediatrics*, 118: e1428–35.

Labree, W., Van de Mheen, H., Rutten, F., Rodenburg, G., Koopmans, G. and Foets, M. (2011) 'Differences in overweight and obesity among children from migrant and native origin: a systematic review of the European literature', *Obesity Reviews*, 1, 12(5): e535–47.

Liu, B., Jorm, L. and Banks, E. (2010) **'**Parity, breastfeeding, and the subsequent risk of maternal type 2 diabetes', *Diabetes Care*, 33 (6): 1239–41.

MacLachlan, M. (2006) *Culture and health: A critical perspective towards global health* (2nd edn), Chichester: Wiley.

McAndrew, F., Thompson, J., Fellows, L., Large, A., Speed, M. and Renfrew, M. (2012) 'Infant Feeding Survey 2010', London: Health and Social Care Information Centre, http://content.digital.nhs.uk/catalogue/PUB08694/Infant-Feeding-Survey-2010-Consolidated-Report.pdf

McFadden, A., Renfrew, M. and Atkin, K. (2012) 'Does cultural context make a difference to women's experiences of maternity care? A qualitative study comparing the perspectives of breast-feeding women of Bangladeshi origin and health practitioners', *Health Expectations*, 16(4): e124–35.

McKay, S., Craw, M. and Chopra, D. (2006) *Migrant workers in England and Wales: an assessment of migrant worker health and safety risks*, London: Health and Safety Executive.

Migration Watch UK (2016) '10 Key Points on mass immigration and population growth', https://www.migrationwatchuk.org/briefing-paper/377

Modood, T., Berthoud, R., Lakey, J., Nazroo, J., Smith, P. and Virdee S. (1997) *Ethnic minorities in Britain: Diversity and disadvantage*, London: Policy Studies Institute.

Netto, G., Sosenko, F. and Bramley, G. (2011) *A review of poverty and ethnicity in Scotland*, York: Joseph Rowntree Foundation.

NICE (2008) '*Maternal and child nutrition*', *Public health guideline* [PH11], www.nice.org.uk/guidance/PH11

Nielsen, S. and Krasnik, A. (2010) 'Poorer self-perceived health among migrants and ethnic minorities versus the majority population in Europe: a systematic review', *International Journal of Public Health*, 55(5): 357–71.

Northstone, K., Emmett, P. and Nethersole, F. (2001) 'The effect of age of introduction to lumpy solids on foods eaten and reported feeding difficulties at 6 and 15 months', *Journal of Human Nutrition and Dietetics*, 14: 43–54.

ONS (2016a) 'Population of the UK by country of birth and nationality: 2015', https://www.ons.gov.uk/peoplepopulationandcommunity/populationandmigration/internationalmigration/bulletins/ukpopulationbycountryofbirthandnationality/august2016

ONS (2016b) 'International immigration and the labour market: 2015', https://www.ons.gov.uk/peoplepopulationandcommunity/populationandmigration/internationalmigration/articles/migrationandthelabourmarketuk/2016

ONS (2016c) 'Statistical bulletin: Parents' country of birth, England and Wales: 2015', https://www.ons.gov.uk/peoplepopulationandcommunity/birthsdeathsandmarriages/livebirths/bulletins/parentscountryofbirthenglandandwales/2015#main-points

Pemberton, S., Phillimore, J. and Robinson, D. (2014) 'Causes and experiences of poverty among economic migrants in the UK', IRiS Working Paper Series, no. 4/2014, Birmingham: University of Birmingham.

Perry, J. (2012) 'UK migrants and the private rented sector', Joseph Rowntree Foundation, https://www.jrf.org.uk/report/uk-migrants-and-private-rented-sector

Rechel, B., Mladovsky, P., Ingleby, D., Mackenbach, J. and McKee, M. (2013) 'Migration and health in an increasingly diverse Europe', *The Lancet*, 381 (9873): 1235–45.

Renzaho, A., Swinburn, B. and Burns, C. (2008) 'Maintenance of traditional cultural orientation is associated with lower rates of obesity and sedentary behaviours among African migrant children to Australia', *International Journal of Obesity*, 32(4): 594–600.

Rienzo, C. (2017) 'Briefing: Characteristics and outcomes of migrants in the UK labour market', The Migration Observatory, www.migrationobservatory.ox.ac.uk/briefings/characteristics-and-outcomes-migrants-uk-labour-market

Rutter, J. (2015) *Moving up and getting on: Migration, integration and social cohesion in the UK*, Bristol: Policy Press.

Sanou, D., O'Reilly, E., Ngnie-Teta, I., Batal, M., Mondain, N., Andrew, C., Newbold, B. and Bourgeault, I. (2014) 'Acculturation and nutritional health of immigrants in Canada: a scoping review', *Journal of Immigrant and Minority Health*, 16(1): 24–34.

Schmied, V., Olley, H., Burns, E., Duff, M., Dennis, C. and Dahlen, H. (2012) 'Contradictions and conflict: a meta-ethnographic study of migrant women's experience of breastfeeding in a new country', *BMC Pregnancy and Childbirth*, 12: 163.

Spector, R. (2010) *Cultural diversity in health and illness*, London: Pearson Education International.

Sussner, K., Lindsay, A. and Peterson, K. (2008) 'The influence of acculturation on breastfeeding initiation and duration in low income women in the US', *Journal of Biosocial Science*, 40 (05): 673–96.

United Nations (2015) 'International migrant stock, 2015', www.un.org/en/development/desa/population/migration/data/estimates2/estimates15.shtml

United Nations Statistical Commission (1998) 'Recommendations for the 2000 censuses of population and housing in the ECE region, Statistical standards and studies – No. 49', www.unece.org/fileadmin/DAM/stats/documents/statistical_standards_&_studies/49.e.pdf

Van Cleemput P. and Parry G. (2001) 'Health status of Gypsy Travellers', *Journal of Public Health*, 23(2): 129–134.

Vargas-Silva, C. and Markaki, Y. (2017) 'Briefing (5th revision): EU migration to and from the UK', The Migration Observatory, www.migrationobservatory.ox.ac.uk/resources/briefings/eu-migration-to-and-from-the-uk

Wallby, T., Lagerberg, D. and Magnusson, M. (2017) 'Relationship between breastfeeding and early childhood obesity: results of a prospective longitudinal study from birth to four Years', *Breastfeeding Medicine*, 12(1): 48–53.

WHO (2003) 'Global strategy for infant and young child feeding, Geneva: World Health Organisation', www.who.int/nutrition/publications/gs_infant_feeding_text_eng.pdf

SIX

Changing cultures of night-time breastfeeding and sleep in the US

Cecilia Tomori

Introduction

Expectant parents in the US usually receive advice on all aspects of pregnancy, childbirth and infant care from multiple medical experts. This guidance reflects cultural assumptions that childbearing requires specialised medical knowledge, which divides the care of mothers and infants under the supervision of separate medical experts, and further fragments various aspects of infant care, including feeding and sleep. This chapter uses historical and ethnographic research to explore the origins of these assumptions and their consequences for American parents who embark on breastfeeding. I suggest that severing the links between these evolutionarily and physiologically connected domains (McKenna et al, 2007; McKenna and Gettler, 2016) has had a significant detrimental impact on night-time infant care. Parents have been left without adequate community cultural knowledge about the interaction of breastfeeding and sleep, and assume that these processes are separate. As a result, they are frequently surprised by infants' night-time behaviour and have difficulties navigating night-time breastfeeding and sleep. These challenges constitute an important element of an already formidable set of barriers to breastfeeding in the United States, where structural support is extremely limited and breastfeeding remains a controversial practice (Tomori et al, 2016). The anthropological lessons from this chapter can be used to make breastfeeding more feasible and sustainable for all families, by developing integrative models that support the dynamic interactions between mothers and infants throughout the day and night.

The origins of fragmentation

The medicalisation of childbirth and the decline of breastfeeding

In colonial America, midwives attended women and their families throughout the entire circle of life from birth to death. Midwives supported the full spectrum of childbearing by assisting during labour and birthing, helping mothers learn to breastfeed, care for their infants and deal with breastfeeding difficulties. All of these events took place in the family home, with the midwife travelling to her charges as she was needed in the community. The rhythm of this life is apparent in Ulrich's (1990) masterful study of Martha Ballard, a midwife living in Maine during the 1700s and early 1800s, who left behind a detailed diary of her daily activities. Ballard travelled throughout the day or night, sometimes in trying weather conditions, on foot, horseback and even by canoe, to attend women in childbirth and to carry out her other duties.

Ballard's brief reports of her midwifery work include multiple challenges ranging from difficult births to breastfeeding problems, such as breast infections. Notably absent from these accounts, however, are concerns about infant feeding decisions, the frequency of infant feeding or infant sleep. During this time, most women breastfed their infants in response to their infants' needs throughout the day and night. From the 17th century to the middle of the 19th century, medical advice in Europe and the US reflected this responsive attitude, by encouraging women to simply feed their babies: 'As to the time and hour it needs no limits, for it may be at any time, night or day, when he hath a mind' (Salmon, 1994: 256). Any concerns presented in the medical literature during this period tend to address wealthier women's childbearing difficulties, which is a topic in its own right that I will not delve into here. Most Euro-American families slept within arm's reach of their infants, who were usually in a cradle, and mothers could easily breastfeed their infants during the night as needed. The relatively limited attention to infant sleep compared to other aspects of infant care, and the portrayal of infant sleep as an activity that took place with ease, indicate that infant sleep was simply not considered particularly problematic during this time (Stearns et al , 1996).

The end of the 19th century, however, gave rise to dramatic transformations in American childbearing practices. Elite women began to invite male physicians into their homes to attend them in childbirth, tempted by promises of new kinds of pain relief (Leavitt, 1988). Physician-attended childbirth became increasingly fashionable among middle-class women as well. The increased need for supervision prompted by the growing popularity of anaesthesia and the development of new surgical techniques led to childbirth being brought into the hospital (Leavitt, 1988). Upper-class white women also led the way in seeking out other new and 'modern' parenting practices. As with childbirth, these practices then became templates for middle-class women to emulate, and they were transformed into standards that were often more forcefully dictated to poor and racial/ ethnic minority women. For instance, physicians actively sought to discredit midwives and older relatives as sources of knowledge by portraying them as ignorant and 'backward', as they sought to gain greater control over childbearing and infant care (Leavitt, 1988; Fraser, 1998). By the middle of the 20th century, the medicalisation of childbirth was complete. Whereas in the 19th century nearly all women were attended by midwives in their homes, by the 1950s 80% of women gave birth at hospitals overseen by physicians and teams of nurses (Leavitt, 1988).

These key transformations of childbearing practices were facilitated by other large-scale social changes. Factory labour became more common than agricultural routines, which were often more amenable to children's presence. Migration of people to cities eroded the communities of knowledge and care on which childbearing women traditionally relied. Romantic love and sexual partnership became valued over childrearing in marriage (Wolf, 2001). Novel ideas about time, which emerged with the role of the clock in factory labour (Thompson, 1967), increasingly spread to other domains of life, including childbearing and infant care. The growing dominance of scientific thinking that was associated with ideas of progress and modernity added further emphasis to measurability and regularity in everyday life (Apple, 1987; Millard, 1990).

Unfortunately, early hospital care did not necessarily improve birth outcomes for women and children, and had profoundly detrimental effects on breastfeeding (Apple, 1987; Leavitt, 1988). Hospital wards provided a new environment for the rapid spread of infections, which was not successfully addressed until the introduction of antibiotics in the mid-20th century. Misguided attempts at infection control were a key driving force behind a number of hospital procedures that limited contact between mothers and babies, and consequently undermined breastfeeding (Apple, 1987; Leavitt, 1988). Additionally, women often underwent interventions in hospital births, such as anaesthesia or strong pain killers, which limited their awareness of the process and had an adverse impact on babies' abilities to latch and initiate breastfeeding

(Apple, 1987; Leavitt, 1988). Mothers and babies were frequently separated for many hours after the birth as they both recovered from the interventions, and were only given the opportunity to feed every few hours. Lengthy intervals between feedings and limited time on the breast made establishing breastfeeding difficult, if not impossible. Many women also received injections or pills to dry up their milk regardless of their desires because hospital staff considered breastfeeding-related care burdensome. Even if they did breastfeed at the hospital, babies might be given infant formula when they were separated from their mothers in the hospital nursery. As more women gave birth in hospitals throughout the twentieth century, hospitals became a locus where physicians consolidated their authority over childbirth and where the medicalisation and fragmentation of maternal and infant care became routine and normalised.

Infant formulas offered a perfect fit for the kind of scientific thinking and routines implemented by hospitals (Apple, 1987). Infant formulas were initially created by physicians as an emergency measure for situations when a mother was unable to breastfeed and another lactating woman could not be found to breastfeed the infant. While physicians recognised that breast milk substitutes carried numerous risks, they also found aspects of this innovation appealing. The components used to make infant formula could be precisely measured, combined in predictable, consistent proportions, and given to babies through feeding bottles. This gave caregivers the opportunity to provide infants with precise amounts of food at regular intervals measured by the clock, in accordance with medical recommendations (Apple, 1987; Millard, 1990). Even greater precision and standardisation could be achieved with the rise of the industrial production of infant formulas based on cow's milk. This kind of regimented infant food delivery system, which involved measurement and documentation, suited the factory-style hospital routines carried out by nursing staff that were regulated by the clock. These institutional routines could then be carried out of the hospital and into the home once mothers and infants were discharged.

Commercial infant formulas were popularised by the rise of advertising, often directly evoking medical authority to endorse products. Early advertising dating back to the end of the 19th and beginning of the 20th century often featured images of chubby, smiling infants who were fed a particular brand of infant formula. The adverts usually claimed that health benefits could be achieved from using the product, sometimes by juxtaposing the chubby child with another, smaller child who was considered less fortunate because she did not receive this manufactured food (Apple, 1987). Along with commercial infant formulas, parents were also targeted with intensive advertising for commercial baby foods (Bentley, 2014). Consequently, while at the turn of the century most mothers did not give solid food to their infants until they were six months or older, by the 1950s the infant food industry (greatly aided by physicians) had convinced parents that babies were ready for and would benefit from these foods as early as just a few weeks old (Bentley, 2014). Breastfeeding was increasingly displaced from both ends – at initiation by hospital routines and the pervasive use of infant formulas, and by the introduction of solid foods in the early months of life.

With all of these different forces combined, it is no wonder that breastfeeding became nearly extinct in American culture by the middle of the twentieth century. In 1948, only 38% of mothers were breastfeeding at hospital discharge, and by 1951 this had reduced to about 20% of mothers (Apple, 1994). We have little information about the duration of breastfeeding at this time. The lack of breastfeeding persisted for decades, as measured by a survey conducted by Ross Laboratories (an infant formula manufacturer), which in 1970 found that only about 25% of women ever breastfed (Ryan, 1997).

Routines and regulation: the rise of artificial feeding and night-time separation

With the medicalisation of childbirth, infant care also began to receive intense scientific scrutiny. For the first time, experts began to recommend that infants should be placed in separate rooms from parents (Stearns et al, 1996). This was a radical departure from previous routines where most families had infants within arm's reach, and after infancy children usually moved on to sleep in the same room as their siblings. The origins of the recommendation to separate infants and parents remain unclear, but some of the reasoning reflected concerns about sexuality and morality, partly driven by Freudian psychology (Stearns et al, 1996; McKenna et al, 2007).

Many early twentieth-century medical experts systematically undermined breastfeeding and, through their focus on routines and night-time mother–child separation, contributed to the growing fragmentation of infant feeding and infant sleep, even as they ostensibly supported breastfeeding. Luther Emmett Holt, a prominent physician member of the US Child Health Committee, became one of the earliest and most well-known proponents of heavily regulated infant care (Apple, 1987; Stearns et al, 1996). Holt authored a brief manual initially intended for nursery maids who were training at the Babies

Hospital in New York City. The upper-class mothers who hired these maids, however, sought out their own copies, which prompted Holt to author a longer version aimed at mothers. Holt's book *The care and feeding of children: A catechism for the use of mothers and children's nurses* was first published in 1894, and became wildly popular, going through 75 printings by 1920 (Apple, 1987).

The Children's Bureau's *Infant care* pamphlet, first published in 1914, borrowed heavily from Holt's book and thereby further expanded his influence (Bentley, 2014). *Infant care* not only reflected a growing middle-class consensus about childrearing, but influenced and reinforced these ideals (Apple, 1987). The pamphlet was widely distributed through government agencies, which printed five million copies by 1930, and a stunning 34 million copies by 1955. Since each copy of the leaflet was likely used for more than one child, and often shared across families, *Infant care* became an enormously influential publication that engaged an exceptionally broad audience.

In the 1917 edition of his book, Holt recommended that in the first two days infants should only be fed four times at six-hour intervals, with one feed between 6 pm and 6 am (the period he called 'night nursings'), because he claimed that little milk was secreted during this time (Holt, 1917: 46). Thereafter, infants were to be fed seven times per day at three-hour intervals, with two feedings during the night, decreasing to a single night-time feed by the age of four months. At each of these feeds infants were to stay at the breast for 20 minutes maximum. By 7–12 months, all night feeds should be eliminated and infants were only to be breastfed five times per day. With these limitations on the frequency and length of feeds, especially at during night-time hours, it would have been virtually impossible for a mother to meet a growing infant's breastfeeding needs, as regular feeding is crucial to building and sustaining an adequate milk supply (Wambach and Riordan, 2015).

Supplementation with liquids and other foods further undermined any chance of breastfeeding success. Holt recommended that infants should not receive other foods beyond breast milk in the first few months, but he also advised that infants should be given water freely. Moreover, Holt suggested that it was actually better for babies to be fed infant formula at night, rather than being breastfed, as he considered this to be less disruptive for mothers' sleep (assuming that bottle-feeding was carried out by someone other than the mother). These recommendations directly contradicted his praise for breastfeeding elsewhere in his manual.

Holt did not make the connection that such a routine would undermine successful breastfeeding. Instead, he (along with many other contemporaneous experts) turned to concerns about the quality and quantity of milk:

Does the nervous condition of the mother affect the milk?

Very much more than her diet; worry, anxiety, fatigue, household cares, social dissipation, etc. have more than anything else to do with the failure of the modern mother as a nurse. Uncontrolled emotions, grief, excitement, fright, passion, may cause milk to disagree with the child, at times they may excite acute illness, and at other times may cause a sudden and complete disappearance of the milk. (Holt, 1917: 45)

At the first signs of any perceived problems with breastfeeding or milk quality, Holt recommended weaning to infant formulas, whose preparation he described in great detail. Holt's praise for breastfeeding therefore rang hollow, as it was coupled with a lack of knowledge about the process and a simultaneous expectation that breastfeeding would fail and artificial feeding would be required.

Establishing and maintaining night-time separation between mothers and infants was a key part of Holt's advice. Holt included detailed instructions for setting up a nursery for the infant in a separate room that included a crib. As with feeding, Holt believed that regularity was essential in establishing good sleep habits, and he therefore emphasised putting babies to sleep at the same time every day. Moreover, he claimed that by the age of three months, and at most by five months, all infants could go without feeding between 10 pm and 6/7 am. Holt identified night feeding as the primary cause of wakefulness and 'disturbed sleep' (Holt, 1917: 91). If infants cried during the night, they were to be checked on, but as long as they were dry and comfortable, and no other problems were noted, they were to be left. Indeed, if a child cried because of 'temper, habit, or to be indulged' (Holt, 1917: 168), Holt recommended that they were 'to be simply allowed to "cry it out". This often requires an hour, and, in extreme cases, two or three hours. A second struggle will seldom last more than ten or fifteen minutes, and a third will rarely be necessary' (Holt, 1917: 168). He nevertheless cautioned that 'Such discipline is not to be carried out unless one is sure as to the cause of habitual crying' (Holt, 1917: 168).

The behaviourist school of psychology, led by John Watson, took these ideas even further. According to Watson, modern life demanded routines and regulation, and infants needed to be trained to accommodate mothers' chores. Once he turned from his academic background to writing for the popular media, Watson exerted an extraordinary influence on middle-class ideas about childrearing. He was a regular contributor to popular US magazines, including *Harper's*, *Cosmopolitan* and *McCall's*. in the 1920s he wrote a series of articles for *McCall's* that became the foundation of his book *Psychological care of the infant and child* (1928), which was co-authored with his wife Rosalie Rayner Watson (Bigelow and Morris, 2001). Watson advised: 'It is wise to start him on [a regular schedule] when he's tiny; most hospitals will help you work out such a schedule and train the new baby to it for a few days before he goes home' (Watson, quoted in Stearns et al, 1996: 352). Watson's ideas follow Holt's and directly tie in with the routines established by hospitals.

Watson was also famous (or infamous) for his advice on limiting affection for children for fear that they would become overly dependent:

> Let your behavior always be objective and kindly firm. Never hug and kiss them, never let them sit in your lap. If you must, kiss them once on the forehead when they say good night. Shake hands with them in the morning. Give them a pat on the head if they have made an extraordinarily good job of a difficult task. (Watson, quoted in Bigelow and Morris, 2001: 27)

This kind of approach also set the tone of his advice for night-time. He advised that once children were put to bed, with minimal affection or bodily contact, they would not require further attention until the morning. Watson did not believe that children were naturally afraid of the dark, or that they needed human contact to be soothed. Although Watson's advice was controversial and contested even in his own time, his emphasis on regularity and routines both during the day and at night gradually gained prominence in infant care (Stearns et al, 1996).

Subsequent popular experts used a gentler tone, yet the emphasis on routines and regularity persisted (Stearns et al, 1996). Benjamin Spock's *The common sense book of baby and child care*, first published in 1946, became the most popular infant care manual of the twentieth century. Although Spock aimed to reassure parents, he still maintained that infants should sleep through the night without feeding within the first few months of life. By this time, both artificial feeding and night-time separation had become widely accepted social norms, and they would serve as the foundation for generations of parents and medical professionals to come. The emphasis on regulating and 'training' infants, coupled with the recommendation to separate infants from parents at night, ultimately completed the severing of breastfeeding from infant sleep.

Consequences of fragmentation

Medical experts did not simply generate ideas that they then imposed on the public. Rather, their ideas reflected certain strands of cultural ideologies (mostly unconscious assumptions about the world) shared by many others in their time. At the same time, these experts wielded increasing power throughout the course of the twentieth century as their advice came to be accepted as 'authoritative knowledge': knowledge that 'counts' (Jordan, 1997). While upper- and middle-class US women often sought out these experts, they also had growing say over the normative standards applicable for all mothers, including those who may have grown up in communities that had different norms – such as Native American, African American and immigrant mothers. In other words, different forms of knowledge became discounted, and regarded as incorrect and unimportant. This also meant that entire traditions of community-based midwifery were actively undermined, and knowledge about childbirth, breastfeeding and infant care was often eroded or actively displaced, to be ultimately replaced by medical experts (Fraser, 1998).

Since the middle of the twentieth century, significant progress has been made in reversing the decline in breastfeeding. Breastfeeding has once again become a cultural ideal (albeit a contested one) thanks to early grassroots efforts led by the La Leche League, further propelled by other social movements and bolstered by a growing body of biomedical research that demonstrates the beneficial effects of breastfeeding (see Tomori, 2014). According to the most recent data from 2013, over 80% of mothers initiate breastfeeding in the US, 51.8% continue to six months and 30.7% to one year (Centers for Disease Control and Prevention, 2016). Nearly all medical experts stand behind official guidelines that recognise breastfeeding as the optimal form of infant feeding.

Despite these dramatic changes that have led to the return of breastfeeding in the US, legacies of the fragmentation of the birth–breastfeeding–infant sleep nexus remain salient today. Most mothers give birth in hospital, where there are high rates of interventions –

including for the 32% who have caesarian sections – and are usually attended by obstetricians (Centers for Disease Control and Prevention, 2017). Medical experts continue to lack adequate knowledge about breastfeeding or how best to support it, and their level of support directly influences breastfeeding outcomes (Szucs et al, 2009; Ramakrishnan et al, 2014). Pervasive socioeconomic inequality and racism in the US medical system has had particularly devastating effects on communities of colour. Even well-intentioned programmes, such as the Special Supplemental Nutrition Program for Women, Infants and Children (WIC), established in 1972, which aimed to address nutrition problems for the poor, who were disproportionately of colour, sometimes contributed to the erosion of breastfeeding and the expansion of the market for infant formula. For decades, WIC distributed free infant formula and offered limited breastfeeding support, and in doing so greatly contributed to artificial feeding among its target communities (Kent, 2006). Although recent efforts have aimed to reverse the damage (Kaplan and Graff, 2008; Jensen and Labbok, 2011), racial breastfeeding inequities endure today (Bartick et al, 2017).

Separate paediatric guidelines governing infant sleep and infant feeding further reflect the legacy of fragmentation. Infant sleep guidelines are driven primarily by concerns about sudden infant death syndrome (SIDS). These guidelines have assumed that solitary sleep is the norm, while sharing a sleep surface with one's infant is considered 'risky'. Although experts have long suggested that breastfeeding has considerable positive effects on SIDS, it took years of debate before breastfeeding's role in the prevention of SIDS was included in the American Academy of Pediatrics (AAP) infant sleep guidelines (AAP Task Force, 2011; Tomori, 2014). Breastfeeding is still not sufficiently highlighted in the 2016 recommendations, although infants fed with formula milk have twice the risk of SIDS (Moon and AAP Task Force on SIDS, 2016); instead, breastfeeding is listed as just one of many factors that reduce the risk of SIDS. The guidance overlooks the evolutionary significance of breastfeeding as the human species-specific norm for establishing the baseline risk of SIDS. Additionally, there is limited recognition of the physiological interplay between breastfeeding and proximate infant sleep, despite findings that clearly show a close association between breastfeeding and bed sharing (Hauck et al, 2008, 2011; Huang et al, 2013; Ball et al, 2016).

Recommendations against bed sharing remain in place in the most recent updated recommendations from 2016, even though the importance of proximity within the same room is now recognised as an important element of reducing SIDS (Moon and AAP Task Force on SIDS, 2016). In contrast to previous literature (Blair et al, 2014), the AAP's analysis (2016) concluded that bed sharing constitutes an independent source of risk in the absence of other risk factors. The recommendations, however, do not adequately address the potential effects on breastfeeding of the advice against bed sharing.

Books on infant sleep continue to be written by a wealth of expert advisors, including physicians and psychologists, although other self-styled experts have also gained prominence using endorsements from medical practitioners. The emphasis on routines and regularity remains dominant, along with a focus on 'self-soothing' (getting a baby to fall asleep on his or her own) and getting a baby to 'sleep through the night', both of which imply the elimination of night feeds. Most of these experts echo Holt's century-old advice in identifying night waking as a 'sleep problem' that should be eliminated by separating the baby from the caregiver. To accomplish this separation, many parents engage in 'sleep training' – harking back to Watson's advice. This concept relies on various methods to habituate infants to fall asleep on their own in a separate room and to stay there without crying during the period parents define as night-time.

One of the most popular resources for 'sleep training' is Ferber's *Solve your child's sleep problems* (2006). Ferber, just like Holt, identifies night-time feeding as a main cause of infant sleep problems. He recommends disassociating breastfeeding from sleeping, so that infants do not need to breastfeed to go back to sleep. He argues that most night-time feeds are unnecessary and serve to habituate infants to feeding, which causes them to wake: 'This learned hunger then becomes a trigger for extra wakings' (Ferber, 2006: 137). These disruptions are thought to occur more frequently among children under two years of age who are, '*still* breastfeeding or using a bottle' (2006: 137, emphasis mine). Ferber also echoes Holt when he advises that parents should check on infants for safety if they wake 'unnecessarily', but should allow infants to cry on their own so that they 'learn' to sleep through the night. Up until the 1996 edition, Ferber advocated letting infants cry without parental soothing to the point of vomiting, although this was removed from later editions (Tomori, 2014).

The current top hit when searching for 'infant sleep' online – and a bestseller on Amazon's children's health section – is *On becoming babywise: Giving your infant the gift of nighttime sleep*, now in its fifth edition. Although co-author Ezzo is a pastor and has no medical training, the other co-author, Bucknam, is a physician who lends the book medical authority, along with the numerous physician endorsements selected by the publisher. The book advocates establishing a pattern of regular routines, which puts parents in charge of when babies are fed, and encourages them to separate infants spatially and eliminate night-time feedings as quickly as possible. Some statements in an earlier edition virtually replicate Watson's recommendations from the 1920s:

> During the crucial early weeks of stabilization, it is important that you shape and form your baby's routine. Too much flexibility will not allow this to happen. That is why a baby's routine must first be established before flexibility is introduced into baby's day. (Ezzo and Bucknam, 2001)

While the Babywise system advocated by Ezzo and Bucknam has come under scrutiny for unsupported medical claims and interfering with breastfeeding, which could lead to potential underfeeding (Aney, 1998), it remains popular. There are strands of competing advice from other sources that emphasise night-time breastfeeding and proximity, especially from the La Leche League International and proponents of attachment parenting. This advice, however, remains vastly overshadowed by the literature that aims to cultivate solitary sleep. The cornerstone of all the top hits in the baby care/new parent genre is establishing a regular bedtime and night-time routine that limits and ultimately eliminates breastfeeding at night.

The consequences of fragmentation of breastfeeding and infant sleep were apparent in my ethnographic research in the American Midwest (Tomori, 2014). The main foci of childbirth education are labour and birth, which are addressed in several, multi-hour sessions, while the topics of infant care and breastfeeding are usually limited to one session each. Breastfeeding may be mentioned in infant care sessions, usually as an infant feeding choice, but attendance at a separate class is recommended and the subject is therefore left out of sessions on routine infant care. Infant sleep is discussed independently of infant feeding in the infant care sessions. Co-sleeping may be mentioned as a practice that sometimes occurs, but instructors often tiptoe around this topic due to the strong medical recommendations against bed sharing. As a result, parents are unprepared for the realities of navigating breastfeeding and sleep.

My ethnographic findings suggest that parents' expectations are contradicted by their infants' behaviour (Tomori, 2014). Parents were surprised when their infants fell asleep while breastfeeding, woke up when they were put down and seemed to want to breastfeed again. What were they to do? On the one hand, their breastfeeding classes told them that they should breastfeed in response to their baby's needs.

On the other hand, how were they going to get their baby to go to sleep without breastfeeding? And what if the baby only stayed asleep in their arms or when next to their body? Bringing their baby to bed with them might make both breastfeeding and sleep feasible, but medical guidance made them fearful that bed sharing would inadvertently harm their baby. Ultimately, nearly all of the parents brought their infants into bed with them without having planned to do so and continued to bed share to facilitate breastfeeding at least some of the time during the course of the first few months. At the same time, parents also struggled with how to reconcile their bed-sharing practices with cultural norms and expectations. Many parents chose to keep their practice hidden for fear of judgment from relatives and friends, and especially from medical practitioners. While the middle-class, predominately white parents in my study had sufficient educational, socioeconomic, relational and other resources necessary to overcome most breastfeeding barriers, their night-time struggles suggest that the consequences of fragmentation between breastfeeding and sleep could pose significant challenges for most breastfeeding parents.

Conclusion

This chapter explored the historical origins of the fragmentation of birth, breastfeeding and maternal–infant sleep in the US, and its consequences for breastfeeding and sleep. Increased opportunities for medical and commercial interventions in infant feeding and infant sleep arose from the medicalisation of childbirth, the rise of scientific thinking and the erosion of community support along with other social changes. This facilitated the increasing use of artificial feeding, promoted severe limitations on night-time feeding, and advocated the spatial separation of mothers and babies. Together, these changes produced an unprecedented fragmentation of breastfeeding and infant sleep. Although recent decades have seen a return to breastfeeding, the legacies of fragmentation continue to have significant consequences for contemporary parents. Historical and cross-cultural studies can provide a basis for offering better guidance and support for the dynamic day- and night-time interactions between mothers and babies that sustains breastfeeding, sleep and wellbeing.

One such effort, in the UK, is Durham University's Parent-Infant Sleep Lab, which provides evidence-based information for parents and health professionals about human infant sleep using an anthropological perspective. The lab's research has highlighted the misalignments between relatively recent Western cultural practices and the evolutionary context of human infant sleep and feeding behaviour. The lab's educational outreach, via its Infant Sleep Information Source, has transformed parental expectations for night-time infant care and resulted in more appropriate infant sleep guidance in the UK.

This work, which was recently awarded the Queen's Anniversary Prize for Higher Education, could be used as a resource and a model for developing similar approaches in the US and elsewhere.

References

American Academy of Pediatrics Task Force on Sudden Infant Death Syndrome (2011) 'SIDS and other sleep-related infant deaths: expansion of recommendations for a safe infant sleeping environment', *Pediatrics*, 128(5): e1341-e1367.

Aney, M. (1998) '"Babywise" advice linked to dehydration, failure to thrive', *AAP News*, 14(4): 21.

Apple, R. D. (1987) *Mothers and medicine: A social history of infant feeding, 1890–1950*, Madison, WI: University of Wisconsin Press.

Apple, R. D. (1994) 'The medicalization of infant feeding in the United States and New Zealand: two countries, one experience', *Journal of Human Lactation*, 10(1): 31–7.

Ball, H. L., Howel, D., Bryant, A., Best, E., Russell, C. and Ward-Platt, M.(2016) 'Bed-sharing by breastfeeding mothers: who bed-shares and what is the relationship with breastfeeding duration?', *Acta Paediatrica*, 105(6): 628–34.

Bartick, M. C., Jegier, B. J., Green, B. D., Schwartz, E. B., Reinhold, A. G. and Stuebe, A. M. (2017) 'Disparities in breastfeeding: impact on maternal and child health outcomes and costs', *The Journal of Pediatrics*, 181: 49–55.

Bentley, A. (2014) *Inventing baby food: Taste, health, and the industrialization of the American diet*, Berkeley, CA: University of California Press.

Bigelow, K. M. and Morris, E. K. (2001) 'John B. Watson's advice on child rearing: some historical context', *Behavioral Development Bulletin*, 10(1): 26.

Blair, P. S., Sidebotham, P., Pease, A. and Fleming, P. J. (2014) 'Bed-sharing in the absence of hazardous circumstances: is there a risk of sudden infant death syndrome? an analysis from two case-control studies conducted in the UK', *PLoS One*, 9(9): e107799.

Centers for Disease Control and Prevention (2016) 'Breastfeeding among U.S. children born 2002–2013', CDC National Immunization Surveys, www.cdc.gov/breastfeeding/data/nis_data/index.htm

Centers for Disease Control and Prevention (2017) 'Births: Method of delivery', https://www.cdc.gov/nchs/fastats/delivery.htm

Ezzo, G. and Bucknam, R. (2001) *On becoming baby wise: The classic reference guide utilized by over 1,000,000 parents worldwide*, Mt Pleasant, SC: Hawks Flight and Association.

Ferber, R. (2006) *Solve your child's sleep problems*, New York: Fireside.

Fraser, G. J. (1998) *African American midwifery in the South: Dialogues of birth, race, and memory*, Cambridge, MA: Harvard University Press.

Hauck, F. R, Signore, C., Fein, S. B. and Raju, T. N. (2008) 'Infant sleeping arrangements and practices during the first year of life', *Pediatrics*, 122, Suppl 2: S113–20.

Hauck, F. R., Thompson, J. M., Tanabe, K. O., Moon, R. Y. and Vanneman M. M. (2011) 'Breastfeeding and the reduced risk of sudden infant death syndrome: a meta-analysis', *Pediatrics*, 128(1): 1–8.

Holt, L. E. (1917) *The care and feeding of children: A catechism for the use of mothers and children's nurses*, New York and London: D. Appleton.

Huang, Y., Hauck, F. R., Signore, C., Yu, A., Raju,T.N.K., Huang, T.T-K. and Fein, S. B. (2013) 'Influence of bedsharing activity on breastfeeding duration among US mothers', *JAMA Pediatrics*, 167(11): 1038–44.

Jensen, E. and Labbok, M. (2011) 'Unintended consequences of the WIC formula rebate program on infant feeding outcomes: will the new food packages be enough?', *Breastfeeding Medicine*, 6(3): 145–9.

Jordan, B. (1997) 'Authoritative knowledge and its construction', in R. Davis-Floyd and C. F. Sargent (eds) *Childbirth and authoritative knowledge: Cross-cultural perspectives*, Berkeley, CA: University of California Press, pp 55–79.

Kaplan, D. L .and Graff, K. M. (2008) 'Marketing breastfeeding: reversing corporate influence on infant feeding practices', *Journal of Urban Health*, 85(4): 486–504.

Kent, G. (2006) 'WIC's promotion of infant formula in the United States', *International Breastfeeding Journal*, 1(1): 8.

Leavitt, J. W. (1988) *Brought to bed: Childbearing in America, 1750–1950*, New York: Oxford University Press.

McKenna, J. J. and Gettler, L. T. (2016) 'There is no such thing as infant sleep, there is no such thing as breastfeeding, there is only breastsleeping', *Acta Paediatrica*, 105(1): 17–21.

McKenna, J. J., Ball, H. L. and Gettler, L. T. (2007) 'Mother–infant cosleeping, breastfeeding and sudden infant death syndrome: what biological anthropology has discovered about normal infant sleep and pediatric sleep medicine', *American Journal of Physical Anthropology*, 134(S45): 133–161.

Millard, A. V. (1990) 'The place of the clock in pediatric advice: rationales, cultural themes, and impediments to breastfeeding', *Social Science and Medicine*, 31(2): 211–21.

Moon, R. Y. and AAP Task Force On Sudden Infant Death Syndrome (2016) 'SIDS and other sleep-related infant deaths: evidence base for 2016 updated recommendations for a safe infant sleeping environment', *Pediatrics*, 138(5): e20162940.

Ramakrishnan, R., Oberg, C. N. and Kirby, R. S. (2014) 'The association between maternal perception of obstetric and pediatric care providers' attitudes and exclusive breastfeeding outcomes', *Journal of Human Lactation*, 30(1): 80–87.

Ryan, A. S. (1997) 'The resurgence of breastfeeding in the United States', *Pediatrics*, 99(4): e12.

Salmon, M. (1994) 'The cultural significance of breastfeeding and infant care in early modern England and America', *Journal of Social History*, 247(23): 1–15.

Stearns, P. N., Rowland, P. and Giarnella, L. (1996) 'Children's sleep: sketching historical change', *Journal of Social History*, 30(2): 345–66.

Szucs, K. A., Miracle, D. J. and Rosenman, M. B. (2009) 'Breastfeeding knowledge, attitudes, and practices among providers in a medical home', *Breastfeeding Medicine*, 4(1): 31–42.

Thompson, E. P. (1967) 'Time, work-discipline, and industrial capitalism', *Past and Present*, 38(1): 56–97.

Tomori, C. (2014) *Nighttime Breastfeeding: An American cultural dilemma*, New York and London: Berghahn Books.

Tomori, C., Palmquist, A. E. and Dowling, S. (2016) 'Contested moral landscapes: negotiating breastfeeding stigma in breastmilk sharing, nighttime breastfeeding, and long-term breastfeeding in the US and the UK', *Social Science and Medicine*, 168: 178–85.

Ulrich, L. T. (1990) *A midwife's tale: The life of Martha Ballard, based on her diary, 1785–1812*, New York: Vintage.

Wambach, K. and Riordan, J. (2015) *Breastfeeding and human lactation* (5th edn), Burlington, MA: Jones and Bartlett Publishers.

Wolf, J. H. (2001) *Don't kill your baby: Public health and the decline of breastfeeding in the nineteenth and twentieth centuries*, Columbus, OH: Ohio State University Press.

SEVEN

Breastfeeding and modern parenting culture: when worlds collide

Amy Brown

Introduction

The decision to breastfeed or feed with infant formula does not occur in a vacuum. As important as infant feeding decisions are for infant and maternal health, they are but one part of infant care. Modern parents are under considerable pressures. Responsibilities both in the home and in the workplace, coupled with the increasing likelihood of being dispersed from close family, can lead to new mothers feeling overwhelmed by the demands of caring for an infant alone. Many report feeling anxiety, tedium or even regret at their new lives and identities. Caring for newborn infants is often overwhelming; with frequent needs for feeding, comfort and general care, it is not surprising that new mothers can feel overloaded. What was once shared within wider communities, with the support of extended family and likeminded peers, is now often an isolated task.

The combination of maternal isolation and modern lifestyle pressures has paved the way for a multimillion-pound baby care book market, with self-styled experts promising new parents structure to their day, 'control' of their infant and, importantly, time for themselves. Infants, according to these authors, can be trained to feed less frequently, sleep through the night and need little interaction during the day. But what is the evidence base for these books? Do they work? And importantly, what is their impact on mothers and babies? We know that responsive care has the best outcomes for infants – socially, emotionally and educationally. We also know that breastfeeding works best when mothers are responsive, feeding to their infant's cues of hunger and satiety rather than a set routine. Conversely, the pressures on modern parents, and the impact of exhaustion and isolation upon maternal wellbeing, are also clear.

This chapter explores this complex issue by looking at the drivers for parents adopting strict infant routines, alongside the potential impact of this on breastfeeding success. It considers what changes are needed at a societal level to enable both breastfeeding to succeed and maternal wellbeing to be protected.

The transition to motherhood

When a baby is born, so is a mother, and as natural as this process is, this does not mean it is easy, particularly in modern times. The dispersion of families in Western culture means that many younger adults have little experience of caring for infants. In one seminal study of women who had not yet had children, 75% had never held a newborn, while less than 20% had cared for a young baby, for example, by changing a nappy or feeding (Oakley, 1992). For many, the first baby they care for or even hold is their own, and the intensity of this responsibility can come as a shock.

Many new mothers report experiencing significant stress, anxiety and a sense of loss of control during this period (Rossiter, 1998), feeling that they have lost their former lives and identity (Leonard, 1993). It is not uncommon for these feelings to develop into postnatal depression, particularly if a woman's life goals are not primarily centred on family (Salmela-Aro et al, 2001). Symptoms of postnatal depression are reported by one in 10 new mothers (NHS Choices, 2016), with the true figure likely higher, owing to mothers perhaps feeling that they should conceal these emotions. Professional, highly educated women are the most at risk, as they can feel their identity and role has vastly changed (Leigh and Milgrom, 2008).

This transition from independent woman to new mother is a significant period of a woman's life, full of mixed emotions (potentially including grief) as she says goodbye to her old life. Generally, the first months are considered the hardest, with most having made a transition to identifying with the mothering role by the time their baby is three months old (Mercer, 1980). However, not all make this transition so rapidly, and some mothers feel unsettled again when situations change, when their baby is teething, for example, or when returning to work (Rallis et al, 2014).

As part of this transition, a woman will decide how she will mother in terms of what approach she will take. She looks to the beliefs and behaviours of those around her: her own mother, peers or perceived experts. Following an approach by those she trusts or admires can bring confidence (Mercer, 1986). This is the stage where many new mothers start to read advice on infant care, in particular, books that may suggest certain ways of interacting with an infant.

The baby care book market

These growing feelings of pressure, isolation and anxiety have enabled a multimillion selling range of baby care books to emerge. These propose parenting techniques and approaches that supposedly reduce the demands of caring for a newborn infant. Although a variety of publications are available, some of the most popular focus on a parent-led approach to infant care, proposing tips and schedules that urge parents to feed babies at a set parent-led interval, to encourage infants to sleep through the night and not to respond immediately to infant cries (see, for example, Blau and Hogg, 2001; Spock, 2011; Ford, 2012).

The question naturally arises as to the impact of these texts. Do they enable the desired behaviour? If so, what is the effect of this on the infant and mother? The evidence behind these texts is scarce. Starting with the positive, recent research has shown a positive association between mothers finding these books useful and maternal wellbeing (Harries and Brown, 2017). Sleep deprivation and excessive crying can increase risk of postnatal depression (Goyal et al, 2007), which can in turn increase the risk of poor maternal–infant attachment (Brockington et al, 2001). Having a 'difficult' baby who is unsettled is also associated with increased feelings of loss of control or identity (Kurth et al, 2010). Therefore, if these books are successful, the appeal for mothers feeling under pressure to juggle it all, often alone, is clear

However, we also know that responsive parenting, where the needs of the infant are met in a timely, appropriate fashion, is critical for infant development (Landry et al, 2006). Positive attachment, where babies feel secure in the care of a primary caregiver, leads to better outcomes socially, educationally and emotionally (Gaertner et al, 2008). Responding sensitively and promptly to an infant's needs is central to developing a strong attachment relationship (Evans and Porter, 2009). This is now an integral part of the Unicef Baby Friendly Initiative standards for maternity, neonatal, health visiting (UK specialist public health nursing) and children's centre (or equivalent early years community settings) services (see 'UK policy context', earlier in this volume).

Responsive care has a physiological impact. In rats, the more a mother licks and grooms her infant rat, the lower the baby's level of stress activity (Szyf et al, 2005). In human infants, stress hormones drop more quickly after a stressful event among those who are parented responsively (Haley and Stansbury, 2003). Conversely, allowing an infant to cry for an extended period can raise stress hormone levels (Engert et al, 2010), which can programme an infant's immature nervous system to be overstimulated in the long term (Loman and Gunnar, 2010). Meeting the normal needs of an infant in terms of responding to cries for food or comfort is therefore important for both attachment and wellbeing (Malekpour, 2007).

What is normal baby behaviour?

In addition to the importance of responsive care for infants, there is the question of whether adopting the nonresponsive parenting approach recommended in certain baby care books will work. In the research mentioned above, finding these texts useful was associated with greater wellbeing, but only 20% of mothers found they could implement the suggestions in the books, as their infants would not adopt the proposed strict routines. This led to feelings of failure and increased anxiety in over half the sample, with associated higher levels of postnatal depression and with no change in infant behaviour (Harries and Brown, 2017).

Why might the guidance not work? Simply because it is at odds with normal infant needs and behaviour. Infants are programmed to need frequent feeds, to stay close to the caregiver and for their needs to be met throughout a 24-hour period rather than only in the daytime.

Normal breastfeeding frequency

Breastfeeding is the biological norm, with infants programmed to feed frequently (subtle differences occur between breastfeeding and feeding with infant formula, which are considered later in this chapter). Breastfed infants typically feed 8–12 times per 24 hours. Infants most commonly lean towards the latter part of that range, feeding 11–12 times across the 24-hour period (Kent et al, 2006). These feeds don't typically follow a set pattern. Infants feed more frequently before and during a growth spurt, to stimulate additional milk supply (Casiday et al, 2004). Many infants cluster feed, particularly in the evening, where they feed in short bursts over a prolonged period of up to several hours (Frantz, 1985). Additionally, breast milk is not a uniform product. As a feed progresses, fat content increases; fat content and energy density are also higher during the day. This can affect timing and frequency of feeds, as infants receive different concentrations of milk (Khan et al, 2013).

Feeding frequency is also heavily influenced by the Western context. In cultures where co-sleeping and carrying infants in a sling or wrap are common, infants feed far more frequently than this. For example, observational studies of the rural hunter–gatherer tribe known as the !Kung found that infants breastfed on average four times an hour, with most feeds lasting two minutes or less (Konner and Worthman, 1980). Studies carried out among other groups show less frequent feeds but still significantly more than in Western cultures. For example, one study in rural Thailand found that infants averaged 15 feeds over 24 hours (Imong et al, 1989).

Infants need to feed frequently for several reasons. First, their stomach is very small. A typical month-old infant requires around 750 ml of breast milk a day, but has a maximum stomach capacity of 90 ml. Even if they consume until their stomach is full at each feed (which breastfed infants tend not to do), they will still have at least eight breastfeeds in 24 hours (Kent et al, 2006). Second, breast milk is very easily digested because it is low in fat and protein but high in carbohydrates and lactose. So 75% of breastfed infants reach a fasting state within three hours of their last feed; this is quicker than those fed using infant formula (17%) (Tomomasa et al, 1987).

Smaller, more frequent feeds have longer-term benefits for infant weight and appetite regulation. Infants who have larger but less frequent feeds are more likely to be overweight compared to those who feed more frequently (Agras et al, 1987). Infants who feed responsively during the first six months show better appetite control and are less likely to be overweight as toddlers (Brown and Lee, 2012). Frequent feeds are therefore normal and protective of later health.

Normal Infant sleep

Despite common social expectations that infants should sleep through the night once they are a few weeks old, it is common and normal for infants to wake frequently throughout the first year and beyond. Many studies find that between 30 and 80% of infants continue to wake at least once a night during the first year, with the average waking 1.77 times (Hörnell et al, 1999; Brown and Harries, 2015). Waking at night and needing a caregiver to respond is normal for infants, who simply cannot meet their own needs in the way an adult can, and bears no relation to long-term sleep issues (Price et al, 2012).

As well as having frequent needs at night, infants are, from an evolutionary perspective, programmed to want to sleep near their caregivers. Compared to other species, human infants are very vulnerable, being unable to walk until around their first year. This increases their need to be near someone who can care for, protect and meet their needs. In fact, sharing a room or bed with an infant is the predominant global behaviour. One study which explored sleeping habits across 127 different cultural groups found that in 79% of cultures, parents typically slept in the same room as their infant, with 44% sleeping on the same surface (Barry and Paxson, 1971).

Sleeping in the same room as an infant reduces the risk of sudden infant death syndrome (SIDS) by around 50% (Task Force on Sudden Infant Death Syndrome, 2011). Reasons for this include the fact that the room is more likely to be kept at an optimal temperature, increased parental vigilance and greater likelihood of infants being aroused by their parents movements. Infants who die of SIDS are more likely to have had longer periods of uninterrupted sleep and to have moved about less in their sleep, which is thought to be a risk factor for SIDS (Hoppenbrouwers et al, 1982). Sleeping close to the mother is beneficial in other ways too. Infants who sleep close to their mother are more likely to maintain their body temperature (Tuffnell et al, 1996), heart rate (Richard and Mosko, 2004) and have steadier breathing (Richard et al, 1998).

Sleep and breastfeeding are also intertwined (see Chapter Six). From an evolutionary perspective, feeding at night is normal. One study carried out in rural Tanzania found that infants breastfed on average four times a night (Sellen, 2001), while another study in rural Thailand found that as they grew older, infants fed more at night, possibly because they were more active during the day (Imong et al, 1989). Co-sleeping is also associated with a longer breastfeeding duration (Blair and Ball, 2004). To some extent, this may be due to wider parenting style choice: mothers who choose to bed share are also more likely to breastfeed (Ball et al, 2016). However, co-sleeping infants do breastfeed more frequently than infants who sleep separately (McKenna et al, 1997).

The impact of strict routines upon breastfeeding

Given our knowledge of normal infant feeding patterns, and the effects of responsive 24-hour care upon breastfeeding, what is the impact of adopting strict routines for feeding and sleep upon breastfeeding success? Unfortunately, research shows that attempting a strict feeding routine can reduce breast milk supply, increase feeding difficulties and ultimately lead to breastfeeding cessation.

The importance of responsive feeding for breast milk supply

Breast milk supply works predominantly on a demand-and-supply basis. Although milk starts to be produced in small amounts midway through pregnancy, it is the events that occur after delivery that are vital to continued production. The removal of the placenta triggers a rapid increase in milk production, and a rise in prolactin and oxytocin alongside a decrease in oestrogen supports this hormonally (Kent, 2007).

After this initial stage, it is the removal of milk from the breast that is critical for continued breast milk production. The more milk that is removed through the infant feeding or by milk being expressed, the more milk is produced. The female body is adept at matching supply to need. More frequent feeds are associated with greater milk production, while delaying or missing feeds signals to the body that less milk is needed, and the body adjusts accordingly (Wambach and Riordan, 2014).

Feeding responsively whenever a baby signals to be breastfed is therefore critical to breast milk production. When infants are fed responsively, mature milk comes in quicker (Woolridge et al, 1985), they regain their birth weight faster (Illingworth et al, 1952) and the risk of jaundice is lower (Carvalho et al, 1982). Feeding responsively also maintains optimal hormone levels: the more often a baby feeds, the higher the level of prolactin (Tay et al, 1996). Finally, responsive feeding is associated with a reduced occurrence of issues related to breastfeeding discontinuation, such as nipple soreness and engorgement (Brown et al, 2011).

Supplementing with infant formula, particularly in the early days and weeks, can lead to a drop in breast milk supply (Chantry et al, 2014). Likewise, using a dummy (pacifier) can reduce milk intake. One study found that infants who used a dummy spent half an hour less breastfeeding each day, having on average one less feed compared to those who did not use one. The same effect was not found when infants sucked their own fingers, suggesting that there is something about a dummy that distracts an infant from feeding (Aarts et al, 1999).

Responsive feeding is associated with a longer duration of breastfeeding. Mothers who feed responsively are more likely to be exclusively breastfeeding at six weeks (Hörnell et al, 2001). This can be in part explained by greater milk supply. In one experiment conducted in the 1980s, mothers were asked to either feed their baby responsively or feed to a fixed three-to-four-hour schedule. Infants who were fed responsively consumed 30% more milk (De Carvalho et al, 1982).

Research that has explored the impact of attempting to breastfeed to a routine also shows a negative impact on breastfeeding duration. In one study exploring early parenting styles, mothers who used a routine for infant care were less likely to breastfeed at all, but if they did, they were more likely to stop breastfeeding in the early days and weeks (Brown and Arnott, 2014). Likewise, mothers who were concerned about being too nurturing with their infant – that is, they wanted periods of separation – were also less likely to initiate or continue breastfeeding.

In another study, breastfeeding mothers who tried to adopt a strict feeding schedule were more likely to stop compared to those who fed responsively (Brown and Lee, 2013). Attempting to feed to a strict routine is also associated with cessation of breastfeeding for reasons that centre around perceived low milk supply, an unsettled infant and pain – we know these are factors associated with infants not being fed responsively (Brown et al, 2011).

Sleep training can also have a negative impact upon breastfeeding success. An intervention to reduce night waking in babies aged 6–12 months found that rates of breastfeeding fell during the period at a faster rate than would be expected. In part, this could be explained by a significant drop in co-sleeping rates, from 70.1% at the start of the study to 26.1% (Hall et al, 2006). Separating mother and baby in hospital in the early days also leads to lower breastfeeding continuation, likely due to the finding that infants are fed less frequently (Ball et al, 2006).

The appeal of infant formula for those who value a strict routine

The decision to attempt to follow a strict routine rather than breastfeed responsively is therefore a significant risk for low milk supply and breastfeeding cessation. However, a desire to follow an infant routine may also lead mothers to make a conscious decision to use infant formula. While for some a strict routine may require them to stop breastfeeding before they are ready, owing to its impact on milk supply, others may desire a routine and believe that the use of infant formula will enable their baby to regain his or her birth weight faster.

In relation to the transition to motherhood, it is easy to see why books that promise an infant who sleeps through the night and does not need to feed frequently may be appealing, despite the incompatibility with breastfeeding. Many mothers are now caring for their infants in isolation (Paris and Dubus, 2005) and juggle caring for an infant with work, often from when the child is young (Haider et al, 2003; NCT, 2014). In addition, many more mothers than acknowledge it are struggling with postnatal depression (Beck, 2001). The promise of an infant who fits around these demands can seem appealing.

Infant formula use fits more neatly with following a routine for several reasons. First, the same supply issues are not encountered as with breastfeeding. Second, formula-fed infants typically feed less frequently than infants breastfed from the start of life, on average around every three hours (Casiday et al, 2004). Infants fed with formula milk are also more predictable in their feeding pattern, because infant formula is a uniform product (Shealy et al, 2008).

Formula-fed infants typically take in larger amounts of milk per feed than breastfed infants, even in the early days of life. One study found that average intake of milk on day one was 9.6 ml/kg/day for breastfed infants, compared to 18.5 ml/kg/day for other infants. On day two, average intake for breastfed infants was 13 ml/kg/day compared to 42.2 ml/kg/day for the infants fed using infant formula (Dollberget al, 2001). These infants also drink feeds more quickly, consuming over three times more milk per minute than breastfed infants (Paul et al, 1996).

Infants fed using formula milk can also be persuaded to take greater amounts per feed. While breastfed infants need to latch onto the breast using their tongue and jaw to compress the nipple to receive milk, milk is removed from a bottle using a simpler sucking mechanism aided by gravity (Riordan et al, 2005). This means that it is easier to persuade a bottle-fed infant to consume more milk than an infant fed directly from the breast. In one study, when caregivers were told to try to persuade an infant to consume more, milk intake was 10% greater than when they were guided to look for signs of satiety and stopped the feed (Fomon et al, 1964). The potential to persuade the infant to consume more can be appealing for some parents and can directly affect the choice of whether to breastfeed or not. One study found that using a routine to feed was associated with beliefs that infant feeding needed to be convenient, and an increased likelihood of choosing infant formula from birth or stopping breastfeeding after a short duration (Brown et al, 2011).

There is also a common belief that using formula will promote infant sleep. In early infancy this can be true: infants fed this way start sleeping through the night at an earlier age (Ball, 2003). However, once infants are aged 6–12 months, both breastfed and other infants wake at a similar frequency, with most doing so once or twice a night (Brown and Harries, 2015). And low frequency of feeding at night does not necessarily equate with maternal rest time. Despite more frequent feeds, mothers who breastfeed typically get more sleep overall, as the activity duration is shorter (Galbally et al, 2013).

Given the established protection of breastfeeding for maternal and infant health (Ip et al, 2009), and the knowledge that responsive feeding in infancy is important for healthy appetite and weight development (Brown and Lee, 2012), these relationships are concerning. Overwhelmed new parents may be turning to feeding schedules due to sheer exhaustion and time pressures, but this places breastfeeding at risk. Others may choose infant formula because of the perceived control it gives over their infant's routine, to the detriment of infant health. Given that many mothers wish to breastfeed, and that stopping before they are ready can increase risk of feelings of guilt and postnatal depression (Brown et al, 2016), this is concerning.

Conclusion

The increasing demands on new parents can make infant care books that promise to train babies to have fewer needs seem appealing. However, research questions not only their success and impact on infant and maternal wellbeing, but the impact they have on breastfeeding. Routines lead to nonresponsive feeding styles, which can damage milk supply, or the frequent needs of a breastfed baby are viewed as incompatible with achieving a routine. Formula becomes the perceived solution.

Responsive parenting and feeding matters. However, recognising the significant pressures new mothers can face in the early months of infant care is important, particularly if they also return to work or are isolated from close family, leaving them heavily responsible for infant care. These challenges are not insignificant and can contribute to postnatal depression, which in itself can have negative consequences for infant wellbeing and development. A solution that protects both mothers and infants is needed.

Instead of offering infant formula as a solution, we should be investing heavily in practical and emotional support for new families. Motherhood should be valued, with extended, well-paid maternity leave, and high-quality emotional and practical support available for new mothers. Rather than pressurising or forcing mothers to choose between their wellbeing and breastfeeding, we should mother our mothers; give them the care, value and financial support to adopt responsive parenting styles; and promote breastfeeding success. As a society, we need to recognise the importance of the early months, and the return that investing in this period can achieve – for mothers, babies and our future generations.

References

Aarts, C., Hörnell, A., Kylberg, E., Hofvander, Y. and Gebre-Medhin, M. (1999) 'Breastfeeding patterns in relation to thumb sucking and pacifier use', *Pediatrics*, 104(4): e50.

Agras, W. S., Kraemer, H. C., Berkowitz, R. I., Korner, A. F. and Hammer, L. D. (1987) 'Does a vigorous feeding style influence early development of adiposity?', *The Journal of Pediatrics*, 110(5): 799–804.

Ball, H. L. (2003) 'Breastfeeding, bed-sharing, and infant sleep', *Birth*, 30(3): 181–8.

Ball, H. L., Ward-Platt, M. P., Heslop, E., Leech, S. J. and Brown, K. A. (2006) 'Randomised trial of infant sleep location on the postnatal ward', *Archives of Disease in Childhood*, 91(12): 1005–10.

Ball, H. L., Howel, D., Bryant, A., Best, E., Russell, C. and Ward-Platt, M. (2016) 'Bed-sharing by breastfeeding mothers: who bed-shares and what is the relationship with breastfeeding duration?', *Acta Paediatrica*, 105(6): 628–34.

Barr, R. G. and Elias, M. F. (1988) 'Nursing interval and maternal responsivity: effect on early infant crying', *Pediatrics*, 81(4): 529–36.

Barry, H. and Paxson, L. M. (1971), 'Infancy and early childhood: cross-cultural codes 2', Ethnology, 10(4): 466–508.

Beck, C. T. (2001) 'Predictors of postpartum depression: an update', *Nursing Research*, 50(5): 275–85.

Blair, P. S. and Ball, H. L. (2004) 'The prevalence and characteristics associated with parent–infant bed-sharing in England', *Archives of Disease in Childhood*, 89(12): 1106–10.

Blau, M. and Hogg, T. (2001) *Secrets of the baby whisperer: How to calm, connect and communicate with your baby*, Vermilion: London.

Brockington, I. F., Oates, J., George, S., Turner, D., Vostanis, P., Sullivan, M., Loh, C. and Murdoch, C. (2001) 'A screening questionnaire for mother–infant bonding disorders,' *Archives of Women's Mental Health*, 3: 133–140.

Brown, A. and Arnott, B. (2014) 'Breastfeeding duration and early parenting behaviour: the importance of an infant-led, responsive style', *PloS One*, 9(2): e83893.

Brown, A. and Harries, V. (2015) 'Infant sleep and night feeding patterns during later infancy: association with breastfeeding frequency, daytime complementary food intake, and infant weight', *Breastfeeding Medicine*, 10(5): 246–52.

Brown, A. and Lee, M. (2012) 'Breastfeeding during the first year promotes satiety responsiveness in children aged 18–24 months', *Pediatric Obesity*, 7(5): 382–90.

Brown, A. and Lee, M. (2013) 'Breastfeeding is associated with a maternal feeding style low in control from birth', *PloS One*, 8(1): e54229.

Brown, A., Raynor, P. and Lee, M. (2011) 'Maternal control of child-feeding during breast and formula feeding in the first six months post-partum', *Journal of Human Nutrition and Dietetics*, 24(2): 177–86.

Brown, A., Rance, J. and Bennett, P. (2016) 'Understanding the relationship between breastfeeding and postnatal depression: the role of pain and physical difficulties', *Journal of Advanced Nursing*, 72(2): 273–82.

Casiday, R. E., Wright, C. M., Panter-Brick, C. and Parkinson, K. N. (2004) 'Do early infant feeding patterns relate to breast-feeding continuation and weight gain? Data from a longitudinal cohort study', *European Journal of Clinical Nutrition*, 58(9): 1290–6.

Chantry, C. J., Dewey, K. G., Peerson, J. M., Wagner, E. A. and Nommsen-Rivers, L. A. (2014) 'In-hospital formula use increases early breastfeeding cessation among first-time mothers intending to exclusively breastfeed', *The Journal of Pediatrics*, 164(6): 1339–45.

De Carvalho, M., Klaus, M. H. and Merkatz, R. B. (1982) 'Frequency of breast-feeding and serum bilirubin concentration', *American Journal of Diseases of Children*, 136(8): 737–8.

Dollberg, S., Lahav, S. and Mimouni, F. B. (2001) 'A comparison of intakes of breast-fed and bottle-fed infants during the first two days of life', *Journal of the American College of Nutrition*, 20(3): 209–11.

Engert, V., Efanov, S. I., Dedovic, K., Duchesne, A., Dagher, A. and Pruessner, J. C. (2010) 'Perceived early-life maternal care and the cortisol response to repeated psychosocial stress', *Journal of Psychiatry and Neuroscience*, 35: 370–77.

Evans, C. A. and Porter, C. L. (2009) 'The emergence of mother–infant co-regulation during the first year: links to infants' developmental status and attachment', *Infant Behavior and Development*, 32(2): 147–58.

Ford, G. (2012) *Contented little baby book*, London: Random House.

Fomon, S. J., Owen, G. M. and Thomas, L. N. (1964) 'Milk or formula volume ingested by infants fed ad libitum', *American Journal of Diseases of Children*, 108(6): 601–4.

Frantz, K. B. (1991) 'The slow-gaining breastfeeding infant', *NAACOG's Clinical Issues in Perinatal and Women's Health Nursing*, 3(4): 647–55.

Gaertner, B. M., Spinrad, T. L. and Eisenberg, N. (2008) 'Focused attention in toddlers: measurement, stability, and relations to negative emotion and parenting', *Infant and Child Development*, 17(4): 339–63.

Galbally, M., Lewis, A. J., McEgan, K., Scalzo, K. and Islam, F. M. (2013) 'Breastfeeding and infant sleep patterns: an Australian population study', *Journal of Paediatrics and Child Health*, 49(2): e147–52.

Goyal, D., Gay, C. L. and Lee, K. A. (2007) 'Patterns of sleep disruption and depressive symptoms in new mothers', *The Journal of Perinatal and Neonatal nursing*, 21(2): 123–9.

Haider, S. J., Jacknowitz, A. and Schoeni, R. F. (2003) 'Welfare work requirements and child well-being: evidence from the effects on breast-feeding', *Demography*, 40(3): 479–97.

Haley, D. W. and Stansbury, K. (2003) 'Infant stress and parent responsiveness: regulation of physiology and behavior during still-face and reunion', *Child Development*, 74(5): 1534–46.

Hall, W. A., Saunders, R. A., Clauson, M., Carty, E. M. and Janssen, P. A. (2006) 'Effects of an intervention aimed at reducing night waking and signaling in 6- to 12-month-old infants', *Behavioral Sleep Medicine*, 4(4): 242–61.

Harries, V. and Brown, A. (2017). 'The association between use of infant parenting books that promote strict routines, and maternal depression, self-efficacy, and parenting confidence', *Early Child Development and Care*, https://doi.org/10.1080/03004430.2017.13 78650

Hoppenbrouwers, T., Jensen, D., Hodgman, J., Harper, R. and Sterman, M. (1982) 'Body movements during quiet sleep (QS) in subsequent siblings of SIDS', *Clinical Research*, 30(1): A136.

Hörnell, A., Aarts, C., Kylberg, E., Hofvander, Y. and Gebre-Medhin, M. (1999) 'Breastfeeding patterns in exclusively breastfed infants: a longitudinal prospective study in Uppsala, Sweden', *Acta Paediatrica*, 88(2): 203–11.

Hörnell, A., Hofvander, Y. and Kylberg, E. (2001) 'Solids and formula: association with pattern and duration of breastfeeding', *Pediatrics*, 107(3): e38.

Illingworth, R. S. (1952) 'Self-demand feeding', *British Medical Journal*, 2(4798): 1355.

Imong, S. M., Jackson, D. A., Wongsawasdii, L., Ruckphaophunt, S., Tansuhaj, A., Chiowanich, P., Woolridge, M. W., Drewett, R. F., Baum, J. D. and Amatayakul, K. (1989) 'Predictors of breast milk intake in rural northern Thailand', *Journal of Pediatric Gastroenterology and Nutrition*, 8(3): 359–70.

Ip, S., Chung, M., Raman, G., Trikalinos, T. A. and Lau, J. (2009) 'A summary of the Agency for Healthcare Research and Quality's evidence report on breastfeeding in developed countries', *Breastfeeding Medicine*, 4(S1): S-17.

Kent, J. C. (2007) 'How breastfeeding works', *Journal of Midwifery and Women's Health*, 52(6): 564–70.

Kent, J. C., Mitoulas, L. R., Cregan, M. D., Ramsay, D. T., Doherty, D. A. and Hartmann, P. E. (2006) 'Volume and frequency of breastfeedings and fat content of breast milk throughout the day', *Pediatrics*, 117(3): e387–95.

Khan, S., Hepworth, A. R., Prime, D. K., Lai, C. T., Trengove, N. J. and Hartmann, P. E. (2013) 'Variation in fat, lactose, and protein composition in breast milk over 24 hours: associations with infant feeding patterns', *Journal of Human Lactation*, 29(1): 81–9.

Konner, M. and Worthman, C. (1980) 'Nursing frequency, gonadal function, and birth spacing among !Kung hunter-gatherers', *Science*, 207(4432): 788–91.

Kurth, E., Spichiger, E., Cignacco, E., Kennedy, H. P., Glanzmann, R., Schmid, M., Staehelin, K., Schindler, C. and Stutz, E. Z. (2010) 'Predictors of crying problems in the early postpartum period', *Journal of Obstetric, Gynecologic, and Neonatal Nursing*, 39(3): 250–62.

Landry, S. H., Smith, K. E. and Swank, P. R. (2006) 'Responsive parenting: establishing early foundations for social, communication, and independent problem-solving skills', *Developmental Psychology*, 42(4): 627.

Leigh, B. and Milgrom, J. (2008) 'Risk factors for antenatal depression, postnatal depression and parenting stress', *BMC Psychiatry*, 8(1): 24.

Leonard, V. W. (1993) *Stress and coping in the transition to parenthood of first-time mothers with career commitments: An interpretative study*, San Francisco, CA: Department of Nursing, University of California.

Loman, M. M. and Gunnar, M. R. (2010) 'Early experience and the development of stress reactivity and regulation in children', *Neuroscience and Biobehavioral Reviews*, 34(6): 867–76.

Malekpour, M. (2007) 'Effects of attachment on early and later development', *The British Journal of Development Disabilities*, 53(105): 81–95.

McKenna, J. J., Mosko, S. S. and Richard, C. A. (1997) 'Bedsharing promotes breastfeeding', *Pediatrics*, 100(2): 214–19.

Mercer R. T. (1980) 'A theoretical framework for studying factors that impact on the maternal role', *Nursing Research*, 30(2): 73–7.

Mercer, R. T. (1986) *First-time motherhood: Experiences from teens to forties*, New York: Springer.

NCT (2014) *Working it out: New parents' experiences of returning to work*, London: NCT.

NHS Choices (2016) 'Postnatal depression factsheet', www.nhs.uk/conditions/post-natal-depression

Oakley, A. (1992) *Social support and motherhood: the natural history of a research project*, London: Blackwell.

Paris, R. and Dubus, N. (2005) 'Staying connected while nurturing an infant: a challenge of new motherhood', *Family Relations*, 54(1): 72–83.

Paul, K., Dittichová, J. and Papoušek, H. (1996) 'Infant feeding behavior: development in patterns and motivation', *Developmental Psychobiology*, 29(7): 563–76.

Price, A. M., Wake, M., Ukoumunne, O. C. and Hiscock, H. (2012) 'Outcomes at six years of age for children with infant sleep problems: longitudinal community-based study', *Sleep Medicine*, 13(8): 991–8.

Rallis, S., Skouteris, H., McCabe, M. and Milgrom, J. (2014) 'The transition to motherhood: towards a broader understanding of perinatal distress', *Women and Birth*, 27(1): 68–71.

Richard, C. A. and Mosko, S. S. (2004) 'Mother–infant bedsharing is associated with an increase in infant heart rate', Sleep, 27(3): 507–11.

Richard, C. A., Mosko, S. S. and McKenna, J. J. (1998) 'Apnea and periodic breathing in bed-sharing and solitary sleeping infants', *Journal of Applied Physiology*, 84(4): 1374–80.

Riordan, J., Gill-Hopple, K. and Angeron, J. (2005) 'Indicators of effective breastfeeding and estimates of breast milk intake', *Journal of Human Lactation*, 21(4): 406–12.

Rossiter, J. C. (1998), 'Promoting breast feeding: the perceptions of Vietnamese mothers in Sydney, Australia', *Journal of Advanced Nursing*, 28(3): 598–605.

Salmela-Aro, K., Nurmi, J. E., Saisto, T. and Halmesmäki, E. (2001) 'Goal reconstruction and depressive symptoms during the transition to motherhood: evidence from two cross-lagged longitudinal studies', *Journal of Personality and Social Psychology*, 81(6): 1144.

Sellen, D. W. (2001) 'Weaning, complementary feeding, and maternal decision making in a rural East African pastoral population', *Journal of Human Lactation*, 17(3): 233–44.

Shealy, K. R., Scanlon, K. S., Labiner-Wolfe, J., Fein, S. B. and Grummer-Strawn, L. M. (2008) 'Characteristics of breastfeeding practices among US mothers', *Pediatrics*, 122(Supplement 2): S50–5.

Spock, B. (2011) *Dr Spock's baby and child care*, New York: Pocket Books.

Szyf, M., Weaver, I. C., Champagne, F. A., Diorio, J. and Meaney, M. J. (2005) 'Maternal programming of steroid receptor expression and phenotype through DNA methylation in the rat', *Frontiers in Neuroendocrinology*, 26(3): 139–62.

Tomomasa, T., Hyman, P. E., Itoh, K., Hsu, J. Y., Koizumi, T., Itoh, Z. and Kuroume, T. (1987) 'Gastroduodenal motility in neonates: response to human milk compared with cow's milk formula', *Pediatrics*, 80(3): 434–8.

Task Force on Sudden Infant Death Syndrome (2011) 'SIDS and other sleep-related infant deaths: expansion of recommendations for a safe infant sleeping environment', *Pediatrics*, 128: 1030–39.

Tay, C.C.K., Glasier, A. F. and McNeilly, A. S. (1996) 'Twenty-four hour patterns of prolactin secretion during lactation and the relationship to suckling and the resumption of fertility in breast-feeding women', *Human Reproduction*, 11(5): 950–55.

Tuffnell, C. S., Petersen, S. A. and Wailoo, M. P. (1996) 'Higher rectal temperatures in co-sleeping infants', *Archives of Disease in Childhood*, 75(3): 249–50.

Wambach, K. and Riordan, J. (eds) (2014) *Breastfeeding and human lactation*, Burlington, MA: Jones and Bartlett Publishers.

Woolridge, M. W., Greasley, V. and Silpisornkosol, S. (1985) 'The initiation of lactation: the effect of early versus delayed contact for suckling on milk intake in the first week post-partum: a study in Chiang Mai, Northern Thailand', *Early Human Development*, 12(3): 269–78.

EIGHT

Parenting ideologies, infant feeding and popular culture

Abigail Locke

Introduction

Infant feeding is an emotive and politicised topic with various conflicting perspectives. This chapter takes a critical social and health psychological perspective to bring together different strands of the contemporary debate around infant feeding, drawing on ideas across the social and health sciences to explore key points of tension. These include media representation of infant feeding, health promotion discourse in a 'neoliberal' society, and the impact of contemporary parenting ideologies on parenting practices and parenting subjectivities. The aim is to reach a deeper understanding of the ways that competing discourses about what it means to be a 'good parent', and how we feed our infants, become operationalised in these different standpoints, using contemporary examples to illustrate these points of tension.

Infant feeding and the jigsaw of early parenting

To many ordinary people, infant feeding is commonly thought of as a simple choice for mothers to make between breastfeeding their babies or bottle feeding them with infant formula. However, very few people working in the field of infant feeding construct it in such simplistic terms; they recognise the discourses around infant feeding as being both complicated and nuanced. New parents have many decisions to make about the way they will care for their baby, and the way that their babies are fed forms part of the jigsaw of early parenting. One of the points of tension that comes into the infant feeding debates is the emphasis that is placed on *how* to feed babies, and whether it is regarded as just one of the many wide-ranging aspects people must face in the early period of parenting or whether it is the *key* topic of concern above all others.

With the complexities and competing tensions people face during early parenting, it often seems that if something has to give way to ease these tensions, then it is breastfeeding. Some argue that perhaps this has something to do with the wide and easy availability of infant formula. This decision may come about because there is both an alternative way of feeding babies, and because the manufacturing companies market infant formula as a trusted, safe and equal alternative to breast milk (Foss and Southwell, 2006; see Martin et al, 2016, for a recent nutritional comparative analysis of breast and formula milks). Deciding not to breastfeed is highly contentious. It inevitably becomes political. It is emotive for the decision maker and those with whom she interacts. It can be very difficult to talk about, particularly as those mothers who use infant formula to feed their babies might experience shame, guilt and judgment because of their decision-making (Lee, 2007; see also Chapters One and Two in this volume). Breastfeeding can also be problematised, for example, breastfeeding in public (Amir, 2014; Grant, 2016) or breastfeeding for 'too long' (Tomori et al, 2016). Feeding with infant formula has become the 'wet nurse' of some contemporary industrialised cultures, as other forms of support or cultural mechanisms to support breastfeeding may not be in place, or mothers are unwilling or unable to seek help to maintain their breastfeeding. In other Western industrialised societies where there are structural mechanisms and financial supports in place for early parenting – for example, Nordic countries such as Sweden, Norway and Denmark – the breastfeeding rates are particularly high in comparison with the UK; initiation rates are at 98% in Sweden, for example, and 72% continue breastfeeding to six months (Save the Children, 2012), much higher than UK estimates for the same period.

When we review the discussions that take place in public spaces about infant feeding practice and the low breastfeeding rates that are recorded in the UK, they are often couched as explanations of 'choice'. However, others (see, for example, Hausman, 2008; Labbok et al, 2008; Smith et al, 2012) argue that framing breastfeeding as a 'lifestyle choice' is problematic, and instead frame it within a larger discourse of reproductive rights and justice. As this chapter will demonstrate, the framing of infant feeding 'choices' situates breastfeeding within larger neoliberal discourses that permeate much of health promotion and parenting cultures more widely. Andrews and Knaak have recently argued that infant feeding practices need to be considered in the wider context wherein medical and health discourses are 'becoming the primary authorities and moral gatekeepers of contemporary parenthood' (Andrews and Knaak, 2013: 88).

Infant feeding is one of many pieces of the complex jigsaw of early parenting, and the formation of this jigsaw starts very early, often in the antenatal period when women are starting to prepare themselves for motherhood. The jigsaw pieces include things like what kind of birth a woman is expecting and the kind of birth she has, where the baby sleeps in the night-time and whether a mother is able to/or wants to wear her baby in a sling or push her baby in a buggy/stroller when she is out in the world and away from home. If a mother is economically active in paid employment, it will also include what type of maternity leave provision is available and/or whether parental leave may be shared with her partner, as well as who else may be available to care for the baby and whether the mother wants them to or not. If we are truly to gain some insight into how and why the current infant feeding decisions are made by mothers, then an understanding of these issues needs to be reached in situ.

The decisions that are made by mothers around infant feeding practices demonstrate a culture of parenting which is built around a discourse of 'good mothering' (Lee, 2008; Knaak, 2010; Andrews and Knaak, 2013; Locke, 2015). This makes the promotion of breastfeeding problematic and emotionally charged, because of the values associated with good mothering (see Chapters One and Two). It also raises the possibility that the situation is being framed by neoliberal discourses where breastfeeding is being promoted as an example of 'good mothering' to women who, for a variety of reasons, may not perceive themselves as having a full choice in their infant feeding decisions, and therefore struggle to be positioned as 'good mothers' within this discourse. If this is the case, then we need to explore what alternatives are available to policy makers so that we may promote breastfeeding in such a way as to encourage but not alienate the women who do not breastfeed their babies past the age of six weeks (McAndrew et al, 2012). It raises the challenge of how we may arrive at a situation like that in Scandinavian countries where breastfeeding babies is the norm, when it is not currently the case in the UK or the US.

Difficult decisions face health professionals and policy makers about whether the main focus should be on the promotion of breastfeeding in and of itself when there is such a large reduction in mothers who initiate breastfeeding and mothers who continue to breastfeed beyond a few weeks. I wish to argue that we should be looking at what happens in those initial days and weeks after childbirth, in order to reach a greater understanding of the reasons why women stop breastfeeding and switch to feeding their babies infant formula. The focus of our enquiry should be on how women resolve these competing tensions as they negotiate their way through early parenthood. To help contextualise the debates, the chapter will now move on to consider contemporary ideologies and parenting cultures.

Considering the scene in current infant feeding debates

For many commentators, the 'choice' of infant feeding method has gone beyond the practice of feeding babies. It has become inextricably linked to cultures of motherhood and displays of (good) mothering practice, and infused with moral statements and judgment (Knaak, 2010; Faircloth, 2013). This may be an unintended result of the breastfeeding advocacy of the past couple of decades, commonly illustrated by the message 'breast is best'. In this section I will explore how this becomes interpreted by wider societal discourses around mothering, and look at what the effects are on those mothers who for whatever reason do not initiate breastfeeding or continue to breastfeed beyond the early days.

As has been widely noted (see, for example, Phoenix and Woollett, 1991; Knaak, 2010), the ideology of 'good mothering' is fraught with many different assumptions about what it is that we are referring to. For some writers, this idealised version of the good mother is typically middle class, and often a stay-at-home mother, who is positioned as fulfilled through her domesticity (Johnston and Swanson, 2006). Clearly, this is problematic, as it excludes whole swathes of women from the picture, and as Byrne claims: 'at the core of practices of motherhood lies the intersection of race, class and gender, with white middle-classness often functioning as a norm of motherhood' (Byrne, 2006: 1002). A consequence of this idealised good mother ideology is that working-class mothers are marginalised and excluded, and their parenting practices made invisible (Gillies, 2007), while middle-class mothers' engagement with raising their children as a kind of parenting 'project' is portrayed as the norm. We can see such a portrayal in the following extract from the *Guardian* newspaper discussing parenting and contemporary parenting cultures in the UK:

> Anyone currently caught up in the maelstrom of parenting a small child in the UK will be acquainted with the shibboleths of contemporary maternal culture: 'natural pregnancy', 'natural birth', postpartum bonding fostered by 'plenty of skin-to-skin contact', 'baby-led weaning', 'baby-wearing', 'co-sleeping' and, above all, on-demand breastfeeding at least until the age of two, as recommended

by the World Health Organization. It takes a lot of nerve
for a new mother to defy these recommendations. (Hewitt,
2013)

This gives a flavour of what contemporary idealised maternal culture
is thought to be, highlighting naturalness, baby-led mothering practice
and acting in such a way as to maximise the future potential of the baby
as she grows into childhood and beyond (Sears and Sears, 2001). While
the article notes that it takes a 'lot of nerve' to go against this current, it
serves to demonstrate how contemporary maternal culture constructs
'good motherhood'. However, the intersectional differences that
constitute good motherhood need greater consideration in the context
of infant feeding in the UK, so that we are able to consider context-
dependent ways of promoting healthy practices. From the *Guardian*
example, we can start to see how the notion of the 'good mother' has
been constructed, and how certain practices of mothering are privileged
for inclusion in this debate while others remain invisible and are simply
not considered. We can also see how the media constructs breastfeeding
as part of this good mothering discourse, tying it in with the global
health message of the World Health Organization that 'breast is best'.
While this is part of a dominant discourse around good mothering,
this message may be resisted in some quarters and other forms of good
motherhood may become constructed (Murphy, 1999) – perhaps this
accounts for the differing rates of breastfeeding uptake across different
socio-economic groups. Tied up with the 'breast is best' promotion
over the past couple of decades is the shame and guilt that women who
have not breastfed might experience (Lee, 2007; see also Chapters One
and Two in this volume). For us to build a more nuanced model of
good mothering, it is important that we consider how these cultures
are intersecting with infant feeding decisions.

Hays (1996) introduces us to the concept of 'intensive' motherhood
and the associated tensions women experience between trying to
be both the good mother and the successful citizen. She notes that
mothering in contemporary society has become defined by women
being overwhelmingly child-centred and self-sacrificial in their
everyday lives. This concept has been picked up and elaborated by
more recent commentators on motherhood who have described it
similarly as 'overzealous motherhood' (Badinter, 2012) and 'total
motherhood' (Wolf, 2007, 2011). Women who do not or cannot
live up to this idealised form of motherhood may come to fear the
judgement and accusations of others of being a 'bad' mother (Arendell,
2000; Christopher, 2012), whilst those who do adopt these idealised

'markers' of mothering practice, may embrace the superior identity of being the 'good mother' (Hays, 1996).

There are several issues surrounding the ideology, cultural prescriptions and expectations of motherhood that are linked to the choice of infant feeding method. Wolf (2007, 2011) argues that breastfeeding has become tied up with a risk culture, and that some women have responded in a way that she describes as 'total motherhood'. Women's breastfeeding decisions and infant feeding practices have become shrouded in the neoliberal terms of informed choice and risk, and the challenge to their decisions about which methods of feeding to follow are based on parenting ideologies and neoliberal discourses. The essence of Wolf's argument is that infant feeding practices have become bound up with 'good mothering' displays as well as being reinforced by health advocacy messages, and as a result those women who do not breastfeed are open to judgment in a 'total motherhood' culture.

The argument put forward is that mothers who 'choose' not to breastfeed their babies when they have been informed of the associated benefits and risks, display a move against good mothering, because they have not made a decision that is best for their baby or themselves. For Wolf, this kind of reasoning demonstrates how 'total motherhood' has become a pervasive part of infant feeding discourse and debate. Wall (2001) looked at the moral constructions of breastfeeding in health service provider information given out to pregnant women and new mothers in Canada. She noted that running throughout the information given to women was a discourse of attachment and connection that could be realised only through breastfeeding, which was coupled with a medical discourse relating to the benefits of breastfeeding for children's health. Murphy (1999), in her classic study on infant feeding in the UK, also noted the moral accountability that was bound up with infant feeding, in particular, how bottle feeding with infant formula may be seen as the mother acting out some form of model of deviance against the dominant view of 'breast is best'. In her UK-based longitudinal study, Murphy noted that for the mothers who didn't breastfeed, this became not only moral deviance but also a form of resistance. She has further laid out the moral attributes around infant feeding, and how breastfeeding and feeding infant formula are seen to be in a binary opposition relationship (Murphy, 1999, 2000) (see Table 3).

Table 3: Binary opposition of moral attributes around infant feeding

Good	Bad
Breast	Infant formula
Natural	Artificial
Self-sacrificial	Selfish
Responsible	Irresponsible
Health-enhancing	Health-compromising
Benefits	Disadvantages
Caring	Negligent

This notion of resistance can also be seen in the rhetoric that is used in breastfeeding advocacy. Hausman (2008) makes a case for this when she argues that while the arguments around breastfeeding have moved on and developed, the rhetoric used in breastfeeding advocacy draws on older ideas. As a result of this lack of movement, the rhetoric used is not enabling a more diverse set of women to come to a decision to breastfeed; instead, it may be reinforcing divisions by creating a kind of cultural resistance around breastfeeding.

Feminism, choice and infant feeding

Contemporary parenting cultures offer us one lens that we can use to unpack the context in which women make decisions about feeding their babies. Another lens we might use can be borrowed from those on offer by the various forms of feminism. Feminist approaches can demonstrate to us how feminisms and 'choice' may operate within the infant feeding debates, and allow us to understand why some women breastfeed and others do not. Typically, we see feminist writers proposing a set of polarised views of infant feeding that are operating on discourses of rights and choices. The dichotomy of these views can be illustrated in the following statements:

A mother has the right to breastfeed her baby herself in a public setting for as long as she and her baby want or need.

A mother chooses how to feed her baby, whether it be with breast milk from her breast only, expressed breast milk via a bottle only, infant formula only, or a combination of breastfeeding and/or expressed breast milk via a bottle and/or infant formula in her own form of mixed feeding.

Carter (1995) neatly sums up how the competing and mutually antagonistic arguments around infant feeding may be mobilised and reinforced using feminist resources:

> One might see bottle feeding as freeing women from the demands and restrictions of lactation or, on the other hand, as imposed on women by the manufacturers of baby milk depriving them of a unique womanly experience, based on centuries of skill and knowledge. Feminism has been attributed with both these points of view in the infant feeding literature. (Carter, 1995: 14)

Carter offers an analysis of power relations, gender, labour and other issues, and looks at how decisions around infant feeding are made within this wider context. She suggests that for some mothers, feeding their babies using infant formula is a feminist statement. Women who feed their children this way may be seen as not conforming to the hegemonic normative expectations of motherhood, but in doing so are 'expressing various forms of resistance to dominant discourses of femininity within which infant feeding practices are framed' (Carter, 1995: 214). This idea links with what Murphy (1999) found in terms of the cultural resistance to breastfeeding. Similarly, Bartlett (2005) applied a gaze of governmentality to breastfeeding promotion, or 'advocacy rhetoric'. One of the advantages of using this gaze is the illumination of an apparent rhetoric of choice; that women can choose to breastfeed or, indeed, resist this choice. Resisting this dominant choice of breastfeeding can lead women to take up a position of moral deviance, and this advocacy rhetoric may fail if it only focuses on using 'breast is best' as the key message given to women. Using an advocacy rhetoric message of 'breast is best' rests on a presumption that women have a knowledge deficit about the benefits of breastfeeding, including the medical benefits to mothers and babies, and the nutritional aspects. However, typically women know the benefits of breastfeeding, but the continuation rates in the UK remain low nevertheless (see Earle, 2003, for a detailed discussion of this). The rhetorical nature of choice with regard to infant feeding and the 'moral imperative' to breastfeed has also been noted by Crossley (2009). Kelleher points out that 'feminist discussions of breastfeeding offer very little explicit consideration of the physical challenges associated with breastfeeding' (Kelleher, 2006: 2729). At the time of writing, the method of infant feeding is typically constructed as a choice, with breastfeeding seen as the 'informed choice'. However, without cultural enablers and social supports in place, this is not a 'choice' that is open to all new mothers. As Hausman (2008) argues, breastfeeding needs to be framed within a discourse of rights, not constructed notions of informed choices and risks. She claims that formulating breastfeeding in this way would enable more women to breastfeed their babies if they wanted to.

Health promotion and neoliberalism

If we take a look at current health promotion practices, we find that the common discourses are of 'informed choice' and risk. Health promotion takes a position which presumes that, as citizens of a liberal democracy, we make choices about our lives and our health that are based on accurate and true information that we receive from experts or other authority figures via the media or other information sources in order to avoid or minimise the risk of harm to ourselves or our families (Ayo, 2012). These seemingly innocuous ideas of informed choice and risk work within a neoliberal context which is infused with discourses about moral accountability and deviance. It may be useful to consider infant feeding, in particular, breastfeeding, as an act of 'embodied neoliberalism' (Cairns and Johnston, 2015) in which we recognise the bodily surveillance of the new mother as a gendered practice, while also noting how new mothers are both positioned and positioning themselves in these infant feeding discourses.

Scholars have in the past few decades increasingly turned their attention to the notion of risk (Beck, 1992; Heyman et al, 2010), with some authors (Lupton, 1999) linking society's preoccupation with risk to Foucault's notion of governmentality (Foucault, 1991). The contemporary notion of risk which is at play here is one that serves to observe, monitor and contribute to the surveillance of the population by those in power. Central to the theory of governmentality is the idea that within governmental discourses, individuals are positioned as active agents who have the capacity for self-surveillance of their behaviour and the reflexive ability to change their behaviour based on this self-surveillance (Lupton, 1999). Following this line of thought, it is suggested that once individuals are made aware of risk in their lives, they are responsible for taking steps to avoid it, as it is in the best interests of themselves and their families. Underlying this is the idea of rational decision-making, and that people will always make decisions that are in their best interests. As such, individuals are placed in a position where they are accountable for any adverse outcomes they experience by failing to put themselves out of harm's way. The idea is that because people are free rational decision makers and always make decisions that are in their best interests, societies function best with a minimum of state intervention. This neoliberal discourse has become pervasive throughout global North cultures (Phipps, 2014). In this context, the individual can choose their actions but is accountable for those actions and their results, and in the health-promotion frame, the choice is thus characterised as being 'informed'.

Choice is portrayed as a 'central tenet in the women's health movement' (Lippman, 1999: 281) and the drive for autonomy, but these choices, and therefore women's autonomy, are limited through parameters which are set by discussions of risk. Crossley (2009) explores the notion of autonomy and the 'rhetoric of choice' in infant feeding in her account of her own breastfeeding experiences. She notes how her autonomy as a woman is challenged by the experience of the 'moral imperative' to breastfeed that comes through breastfeeding advocacy. These notions of choice and autonomy are at the heart of both postfeminist and neoliberal discourses (Gill, 2006). Key to what Gill defines as a 'post-feminist sensibility' are the ideas of being oneself and pleasing oneself (2006: 153). These are central to a sense of autonomy as a person, which may work to sanction a woman's decision on how to feed her baby. This understanding of autonomy sits against a discussion of costs and benefits (risk discourses) and what may potentially be at stake as a result of this pursuit.

We can speculate that the messages that are broadcast and meant to encourage women to initiate breastfeeding may end up inadvertently being part of a larger kind of cultural resistance to breastfeeding. This resistance to breastfeeding may be deep-rooted in some families, due to many years of feeding practice with infant formula, but it has become bound up with the ways in which good mothering discourses are tied to certain mothering practices and the feeling that mothers have when they do not breastfeed (Grant et al, 2017). The context of decision-making is not always reflected in the advocacy discourses seen in public health campaigns. Consider the following account from a mother about the reasons that she and her peers from her antenatal class stopped breastfeeding (Locke, 2012). This data was drawn from a study that focused on the infant feeding experiences of a number women who all began with the intention of breastfeeding, although some of the sample moved to formula feeding.

> Nobody made that decision. Everybody, every single one
> of them wanted to breastfeed. One girl had, well she had a
> massive baby and a really long labour and really big blood
> loss, so she was anaemic, so her midwife actually said, 'I'm

here to tell you I don't think you should breastfeed.' And it was the best advice she could have heard because she'd have been back in hospital. Somebody else is still combination feeding but she's got postnatal depression and she actually went a bit mental after the birth and just couldn't, you know, produce enough milk because of that and sort of topped it up and has continued to do that. Somebody else's baby was very premature and so it was taking her ages to express and I'm sure that's connected. You know, the baby was in special care and that, you know, it's not conducive to sort of sit there, pumping away in that sort of context, so that was her reason behind it. So you know, every single person had a different, very good reason. It wasn't because they couldn't be bothered or they didn't like the idea or, you know, 'cause they didn't want their baby spoiling their fun bags, it was none of that. It was all about, you know, medical things that happened post birth. (Kath)

In the extract above, Kath is clear to outline the varying reasons that mothers had for stopping breastfeeding. These reasons are founded in medical issues and on their own would potentially have solutions that could result in continued breastfeeding. Note that Kath puts forward the reasons that her antenatal peers stopped breastfeeding, followed by a clear statement that it was not because of a variety of more selfish reasons that are sometimes suggested as reasons that women do not breastfeed, for example, linked to physical appearance. In this sense, then, Kath is orienting to the moral discourses around infant feeding decisions. However, as noted at the beginning of the chapter, infant feeding is one part of the larger jigsaw of early parenting, and as the drop-off in continuation figures demonstrates, it is possible that many women experience infant feeding in this way. Therefore, an understanding of the wider context in which infant feeding decisions are made and continue to be made is an important step in addressing low breastfeeding rates.

Conclusion: putting infant feeding in context

This chapter has discussed some of the complexities in infant feeding decisions, with the aim of contextualising what is often portrayed as a polarised and emotive debate. It has included a discussion of contemporary parenting ideologies, feminisms and infant feeding, before unpacking the way in which neoliberal ideals of 'choice' and 'risk' have become tied up with health promotion messages and breastfeeding advocacy. It argues that some of the complexities and nuances of the infant feeding debates may be one way of explaining discrepancies in rates and the difficulties inherent in breastfeeding promotion strategies.

Some of this stems from the ways in which it is approached – as a topic in its own right or as part of a larger jigsaw of early parenting. The former approach runs the risk of ignoring wider issues that are impacting on infant feeding; the latter runs the risk of downplaying infant feeding methods. These competing tensions appear to be paramount throughout infant feeding and parenting literatures, whichever camp the reader places themselves within.

I would suggest that there needs to be a wider acknowledgment of the mother and her needs. Some research has suggested that mothers can come secondary to the baby in health professional discourses. Fenwick et al (2013), in an examination of the language used by midwives during prenatal sessions, found that language and practices were often limited to convincing women to breastfeed rather than engaging them in conversations that facilitated exploration and discovery of how breastfeeding might be experienced within the mother–infant relationship and broader social/cultural context. Similar research has examined the discourse of midwives around breastfeeding in interactions with breastfeeding mothers (Burns et al, 2012), noting the discourse of breast milk as 'liquid gold'. They argue that this discourse privileges the nutritional aspects of the breast milk over both the practice of breastfeeding and the needs of the mother, leading to an exclusion of communication with and support for the mothers. Obviously, we need to locate these studies in terms of a neoliberal target-driven culture with the wider impacts of austerity and fewer resources.

To end this chapter, I would like to demonstrate how these tensions played out in data that I collected (Locke, 2012). In the following example, a mother, Hayley, having just given birth, and having found it a difficult experience, did not feel that her needs were being recognised. As noted as a point of tension above, it became apparent throughout the interviews that there was a tension between what was considered best for the baby and what was best for the mother with respect to infant feeding, although women were encouraged to persevere with breastfeeding to do what was best for their babies. In the extract below, Hayley tells us about her first experience of breastfeeding after having her baby:

And they'd given me this child, I thought I can't even hold her, and it is drummed into you that it's best for your baby and of course I wanted to pursue it and I know she needed feeding but it did seem really ludicrous for them to be just so focused on that. I remember saying, 'I need a drink,' and they said, 'Yes, we'll get you one soon, just feed the baby first,' and I'm thinking, 'I've just had the worst experience of my life, can I just have a drink please?' (Hayley)

References

Andrews, T. and Knaak, S. (2013) 'Medicalized mothering: experiences with breastfeeding in Canada and Norway', *The Sociological Review*, 61: 88–110.

Amir, L. H. (2014) 'Breastfeeding in public: "you can do it?"', *International Breastfeeding Journal*, 9: 187.

Arendell, T. (2000) 'Conceiving and investigating motherhood: the decade's scholarship', *Journal of Marriage and the Family*, 62: 1192–207.

Ayo, N. (2012) 'Understanding health promotion in a neoliberal climate and the making of health conscious citizens', *Critical Public Health*, 22(1): 99–105.

Badinter, E. (2012) *The conflict: How modern motherhood undermines the status of women*, Translated by Adriana Hunter, New York, NY: Metropolitan Books, Henry Holt and Company.

Bartlett, A. (2005) *Breastwork: Rethinking breastfeeding*, Sydney: University of New South Wales Press.

Beck, U. (1992) *Risk society: Towards a new modernity*, London: Sage.

Burns, E., Schmied, V., Fenwick, J. and Sheehan, A. (2012) 'Liquid gold from the milkbar: constructions of breastmilk and breastfeeding women in the language and practices of midwives', *Social Science and Medicine*, 75: 1737–45.

Byrne, B. (2006) 'In search of a "good mix": class, gender and practices of mothering', *Sociology*, 40(6): 1001–17.

Cairns, K. and Johnston, J. (2015) 'Choosing health: embodied neoliberalism, postfeminism, and the "do-diet"', *Theory and Society*, 44(2): 153–75.

Carter, P. (1995) *Feminism, breasts and breastfeeding*, Basingstoke: Macmillan Press.

Christopher, K. (2012) 'Extensive mothering: employed mothers' constructions of the good mother', *Gender and Society*, 26: 73–96.

Crossley, M. L. (2009) 'Breastfeeding as a moral imperative: an autoethnographic study', *Feminism and Psychology*, 19, 71–87.

Earle, S. (2003) 'Is breast best?: breastfeeding, motherhood and identity', in S. Earle and G. Letherby (eds) *Gender, identity and reproduction: Social perspectives*, London: Palgrave, pp 135–50.

Faircloth, C. (2013) *Militant lactivism? Attachment parenting and intensive motherhood in the UK and France*, Oxford: Berghahn.

Fenwick J., Burns E., Sheehan A. and Schmied V. (2013) 'We only talk about breastfeeding: a discourse analysis of infant feeding messages in antenatal group-based education', *Midwifery*, 29: 425–33.

Foss, K. A. and Southwell, B. G. (2006) 'Infant feeding and the media: the relationship between *Parents' Magazine* content and breastfeeding, 1972–2000,' *International Breastfeeding Journal*, 1: 10.

Foucault, M. (1991) 'Governmentality', in G. Burchell, C. Gordon and P. Miller (eds) *The Foucault effect: Studies in governmentality*, Hemel Hempstead: Harvester Wheatsheaf, pp 87–104.

Gill, R. (2006) *Gender and the media*, Cambridge: Polity Press.

Gillies, V. (2007) *Marginalised mothers: Exploring working-class experiences of parenting*, London: Routledge.

Grant, A. (2016) '"I...don't want to see you flashing your bits around": exhibitionism, othering and good motherhood in online perceptions of public breastfeeding', *Geoforum*, 71: 52–61.

Grant, A., Mannay, D. and Marzella, R. (2017) '"People try and police your behaviour": the impact of surveillance on mothers' and grandmothers' perceptions and experiences of infant feeding', *Families, Relationships and Societies*, https://doi.org/10.1332/204674 317X14888886530223

Hausman, B. (2008) 'Women's liberation and the rhetoric of "choice" in infant feeding debates', *International Breastfeeding Journal*, 3: 10.

Hays, S. (1996) *The cultural contradictions of motherhood*, New Haven, CT: Yale University Press.

Hewitt, R. (2013) '*The Conflict* by Elisabeth Badinter – a review', *The Guardian*, 29 August 2013.

Heyman, B., Alaszewski, A., Shaw, M. and Titterton, M. (2010) *Risk, safety and clinical practice: Health care through the lens of risk*, Oxford: Oxford University Press.

Johnston, D. D. and Swanson, D. H. (2006) 'Constructing the "good mother": the experience of mothering ideologies by work status', *Sex Roles*, 54: 509–19.

Knaak, S. (2010) 'Conceptualising risk, constructing choice: breastfeeding and good mothering in risk society', *Health, Risk and Society*, 12(4): 345–55.

Kelleher, C. M. (2006) 'The physical challenges of early breastfeeding', *Social Science and Medicine*, 63: 2727–38.

Labbok, M., Smith, P. H. and Taylor, E. C. (2008) 'Breastfeeding and feminism: a focus on reproductive health, rights and justice', *International Breastfeeding Journal*, 3: 8.

Lee, E. (2007) 'Health, morality, and infant feeding: British mothers' experiences of formula milk use in the early weeks', *Sociology of Health and Illness*, 29(7): 1075–90.

Lee, E. (2008) 'Living with risk in the age of "intensive motherhood": maternal identity and infant feeding', *Health, Risk and Society*, 10: 467–77.

Lippman, A. (1999) 'Choice as a risk to women's health', *Health, Risk and Society*, 1: 281–91.

Locke, A. (2012) *Tensions, expectations and realistic advice in early breastfeeding,* Conference paper presented at the British Psychological Society Psychology of Women Section PoWS Annual Conference, 11–13 July 2012, Cumberland Lodge, Windsor, UK.

Locke, A. (2015) 'Agency, "good motherhood" and "a load of mush": constructions of baby-led weaning in the press', *Women's Studies International Forum*, 53: 139–46.

Lupton, D. (1999) *Risk*, London: Routledge.

McAndrew, F., Thompson, J., Fellows, L., Large, A., Speed, M. and Renfrew, M. J. (2012) 'Infant Feeding Survey 2010', London: Health and Social Care Information Centre, http://content.digital.nhs.uk/catalogue/PUB08694/Infant-Feeding-Survey-2010-Consolidated-Report.pdf

Martin, C. R., Lin, P.-R. and Blackburn, G. L. (2016) 'Review of infant feeding: key features of breast milk and infant formula', *Nutrients*, 8(5): 279.

Murphy, E. (1999) '"Breast is best": infant feeding and maternal deviance', *Sociology of Health and Illness*, 21: 187–208.

Murphy, E. (2000) 'Risk, responsibility, and rhetoric in infant feeding', *Journal of Contemporary Ethnography*, 29: 291–325.

Phipps, A. (2014) *The politics of the body: Gender in a neoliberal and neoconservative age*, Cambridge: Polity Press.

Phoenix, A. and Woollett, A. (1991) 'Motherhood: social construction, politics and psychology', in A. Phoenix, A. Woollett and E. Lloyd (eds) *Motherhood: Meanings, practices and ideologies*, Thousand Oaks, CA: Sage, pp 13–27.

Save the Children (2012) *Nutrition in the first 1000 days: State of the world's mothers*, London: Save the Children International.

Sears, W. and Sears, M. (2001) *The attachment parenting book: A commonsense guide to understanding and nurturing your baby*, London: Little, Brown and Company.

Smith, P. H., Hausman, B. and Labbok, M. (2012) *Beyond health, beyond choice: Breastfeeding constraints and realities*, New Brunswick, NJ: Rutgers University Press.

Tomori, C. (2015) *Nighttime breastfeeding: An American cultural dilemma*, New York: Berghahn Books.

Tomori, C., Palmquist, A. and Dowling, S. (2016) 'Contested moral landscapes: negotiating breastfeeding stigma in breastmilk sharing, nighttime breastfeeding, and long-term breastfeeding in the US and UK', *Social Science and Medicine*, 168: 178–85.

Wall, G. (2001) 'Moral constructions of motherhood in breastfeeding discourse', *Gender and Society*, 15: 592–610.

Wolf, J. B. (2007) 'Is breast really best? Risk and total motherhood in the national breastfeeding awareness campaign', *Journal of Health, Politics, Policy and Law*, 32: 595–636.

Wolf, J. B. (2011) *Is breast best? Taking on the breastfeeding experts and the new high stakes of motherhood*, New York: NYU Press.

Cultures of breastfeeding: reflections for policy and practice

Sally Tedstone and Geraldine Lucas

As an infant feeding specialist in midwifery practice and a university senior lecturer in midwifery, we have had some very interesting discussions about the work presented in this group of chapters. It has become clear to us that what midwifery students learn is heavily influenced by the practice they observe while on clinical placements. This may seem obvious, but from our perspective the pressures that higher education and the NHS face in the current climate of austerity in the UK have resulted in a squeeze on opportunities for dialogue, feedback and reflection between the two sectors, and we feel that this has a potential impact on the quality of student learning.

Brown's chapter (Chapter Seven) explores the challenges of modern parenting in the UK and how these can impact on a mother's infant feeding journey. Brown has an accessible writing style that provides a useful summary of the context in which professional support for infant feeding is provided. This chapter is thought-provoking and valuable to all who seek to understand the complexity of infant feeding in its social context. Our understanding of the impact of prenatal and very early childhood experiences on infant, child and adult wellbeing has developed rapidly over recent years. We have identified the need to consider what student midwives are learning in this area and how to ensure that practising midwives are updated, in order that new knowledge is embedded into practice. We feel that we should be creating opportunities for student midwives to observe a variety of the healthcare professionals that support pregnant women and new mothers, particularly health visitors (UK public health nurses) who provide a mandated service (NHS England, 2016) starting at 28 weeks of pregnancy and continuing into the early postnatal period and beyond for all mothers in England (with similar services provided in other parts of the UK). We feel there is a need for multi-professional education, so that students can develop an enhanced knowledge in relation to breastfeeding, parenting, infant sleep and behaviour.

Brown's discussion on the transition to motherhood led us to reflect on how student midwives learn about this process. We have observed that without continuity of care, students do not witness a woman's journey into motherhood. The model of midwifery currently used in the healthcare delivery organisations in our local area provides limited continuity of care. However, following the *Better births* report (NHS England, 2016) plans to address this are being developed. Alongside this development, many UK universities are encouraging the use of caseloads as part of clinical learning to expose students to continuity of care.

Condon (Chapter Five) provides midwifery and related professions with a useful insight into the lived infant feeding experiences of parents born abroad who are raising a child in the UK. She describes the changes in infant feeding practices that are often seen in women who relocate, and how a range of disablers such as poverty, poor housing and employment appear to have an impact on breastfeeding. In the context of midwifery education, we feel that midwives need to be aware of women's social circumstances and have insight into the challenges facing migrant mothers. We asked ourselves the question, 'How many midwives have access to the information in Condon's research?' This led us to consider the subtle bias towards valuing medical research above that of social science research which we have observed in midwifery practice.

Condon also draws our attention to wider literature on the experiences of black and minority ethnic women in maternity services, which can lack cultural sensitivity (McFadden et al, 2013). This raises a question for us about how we can address this in practice. In university settings, we think it is important for students to reflect on and find out about their community areas, and subsequently to share their findings within the wider peer group. We know that some students will be exposed to cultural diversity, but others will not, so this might be a positive way to bridge this gap. Condon reports that parents appeared unaware of the implications for the health of mothers and babies of changes in their infant feeding practices adopted since arrival in the UK. This highlights a significant gap in the public health messages received and an opportunity for some collaborative service improvement across maternity and health visiting services.

Locke's work (Chapter Eight) provides us with an insight into some of the discourses that surround infant feeding and parenting. It is challenging to reflect on what this means for midwifery practice, as resonances with the lived experiences of midwives are difficult to identify. To focus on one aspect, Locke argues that women's infant feeding decisions are linked with notions of the 'good' and 'bad' mother, with 'good equals breastfeeding'. This is a complex and deeply personal area. The work of Dyson, who examined factors influencing the infant feeding decision for socioeconomically deprived pregnant teenagers in England, found that 'Breastfeeding was viewed as a morally inappropriate behaviour by most of these teenagers, with formula feeding being perceived as the appropriate behaviour' (Dyson, 2010: 141). Where does this leave us as educators of student and practising midwives? Our aim is simple: to encourage midwives to be aware of the sensitivity of this area, to understand the many different influences on women's lives in order that midwives are truly non-judgmental in their attitudes towards women's decisions. We support midwives to practise in a way that is woman-centred, listening to each individual woman and her questions, concerns, aspirations and goals, and supporting her on her journey.

In the UK, the Unicef UK Baby Friendly Initiative has had a significant influence on improving practice in this area, with over 90% of maternity services working towards or having achieved Baby Friendly accreditation (see 'UK policy context'). These standards require that information given is woman-centred and covers a wider range of topics, including babies' needs for closeness and comfort (Unicef UK, 2013). The woman is the focus of conversations; listening to her thoughts and questions is the starting point. This strategy, when implemented well, allows for a more nuanced approach that understands an individual woman's perspective and concerns and supports her decision-making. This requires excellent communication skills from midwives, and leads us back to reflecting on the central question of what students learn in university, and in practice, and whether the two are aligned and mutually supportive.

The campaigning and advocacy work of the Unicef UK Baby Friendly Initiative is also influencing the wider cultural context in the UK. The 2016 campaign Change the Conversation calls on the UK Government to 'take urgent action to remove the barriers to breastfeeding in the UK' (Unicef, 2016a). One aspect of this campaign is a call to acknowledge the responsibility we have as a society for the low breastfeeding rates, rather than blame individual women, which is an important positive step towards changing the culture.

Both the changes made to the Unicef UK Baby Friendly Initiative standards and the wider advocacy work of the initiative in the UK are informed by the debates and critique presented in Locke's chapter, and aim to move us forward towards a supportive culture where women can make the choices that are right for them and their baby, knowing they will be supported.

Tomori (Chapter Six) provides us with a fascinating exploration of the historical origins of the fragmentation of birth, breastfeeding and maternal–infant sleep. The consequences of the trends Tomori describes have been far-reaching, leaving a legacy of parental anxiety about infant sleep which has implications for feeding choices and maternal wellbeing that are very familiar to our health visitor (public health nursing) colleagues.

Tomori refers to her interesting ethnographic research, which revealed that most parents brought their babies into bed, even though they had not intended to do this because it was 'risky'. This reflects what we know about infant sleep practices in the UK. The work of Helen Ball has brought our attention to night-time parenting practices, through her longitudinal study on parents and infants in the North East of England. Ball found a bed-sharing prevalence of 47–8% among neonates (Ball, 2002). Tomori, referring to her own study, states that 'all parents knew that they should avoid bed sharing because of sudden infant death syndrome (SIDS)'. This led us to reflect on how this particular debate has shifted in the UK. National guidance carefully reflects the evidence base and steers professionals away from outright bans to a discussion of risk (National Institute of Health and Care Excellence [NICE], 2015). Health professionals are supported by several evidence-based information sources, such as *Caring for your baby at night* (Unicef UK, 2016b) the Lullaby Trust website and Durham University's Infant Sleep Information Service.

Discussing what Tomori refers to as the legacies of fragmentation for parents led us back to the topic of parent education. We have experience locally of services which provide evidence-based parent education programmes based on the valuable resource *Preparation for Birth and Beyond* (Department of Health, 2011). Such programmes allow parents the opportunity to gain understanding of the links between early brain development and later life outcomes, and the impact that early life experiences can have on a child's wellbeing. High-quality learning experiences provide an antidote to the medicalisation that Tomori describes. However, quality of services varies considerably and in other local areas fiscal cuts have led to a reduced availability of programmes. We also observe a lack of education opportunities for midwives to update their knowledge on approaches to parent education, and we suspect that there is wide variation in the quality and accessibility of good-quality parent education, certainly in our region of the UK.

Our most significant learning has been the value of connection for our two roles. We have directly experienced the benefits and insight this has brought us, and can see clearly that working more closely together will benefit students and ultimately the parents our services support. Through discussion, we have identified a number of areas where there is a potential issue in that what students are learning in practice may not align with the theoretical knowledge they are taught, particularly at the leading edge of knowledge and practice development. There are identified gaps in practice in supporting parents to transition to parenthood, and collaboration between student midwives and health visitors could bridge this gap, with opportunities for professional development in practice. We need to work with colleagues who have experience in supporting mothers who have migrated to the UK, to develop a quality vision of support and need. We need to learn from Tomori's historical context on medicalisation, and the interplay of other confounding influences, including their impact on breastfeeding. Finally, we need to work with service users so that we continue to embrace woman-centred approaches to care, with acknowledgement that our interactions with women can have a lifelong impact on their experience, and their journeys to parenthood.

References

Ball, H. L. (2002) 'Reasons to bed-share: why parents sleep with their infants', *Journal of Reproductive and Infant Psychology*, 20(4): 207–21.

Department of Health (2011) 'Preparation for birth and beyond: a resource pack for leaders of community groups and activities', Department of Health and Social Care, https://www.gov.uk/government/publications/preparation-for-birth-and-beyond-a-resource-pack-for-leaders-of-community-groups-and-activities

Dyson, L., Green, J. M., Renfrew, M. J., McMillan, B. and Woolridge, M. (2010) 'Factors influencing the infant feeding decision for socioeconomically deprived pregnant teenagers: the moral dimension', *Birth*, 37(2): 141–9.

McFadden, A., Renfrew, M. and Atkin, K. (2013) 'Does cultural context make a difference to women's experiences of maternity care? A qualitative study comparing the perspectives of breast-feeding women of Bangladeshi origin and health practitioners', *Health Expectations*, 16(4): e124–35.

NHS England (2016) 'Better births: Improving outcomes of maternity services in England: A five year forward view for maternity care', https://www.england.nhs.uk/wp-content/uploads/2016/02/national-maternity-review-report.pdf

National Institute of Health and Care Excellence (NICE) (2015) 'Postnatal care quality standard [QS37] Quality statement 4: Infant health – safer infant sleeping', https://www.nice.org.uk/guidance/qs37/chapter/Quality-statement-4-Infant-health-safer-infant-sleeping

Unicef UK (2013) 'Guide to the Baby Friendly Initiative standards', https://www.unicef.org.uk/babyfriendly/baby-friendly-resources/ guidance-for-health-professionals/implementing-the-baby-friendly-standards/guide-to-the-baby-friendly-initiative-standards/

Unicef UK (2016a) 'Join our Change the Conversation campaign', https://www.unicef.org.uk/babyfriendly/baby-friendly-resources/ advocacy/join-our-change-the-conversation-campaign

Unicef UK (2016b) 'Caring for your baby at night', https://www. unicef.org.uk/babyfriendly/baby-friendly-resources/leaflets-and-posters/caring-for-your-baby-at-night

PART III

Breastfeeding and popular culture

NINE

Law of lactation breaks in the UK: employers' perspectives

Melanie Fraser

Introduction

After maternity leave, women who return to work may want to breastfeed or express (pump) breast milk for their baby. These lactation breaks may take place during their working time. Line managers are heavily vested in the process of helping parents manage their new roles and the adjustments that must be made in the return-to-work process. While there is no statutory obligation on UK employers to provide lactation breaks to their staff, the cumulative effect of an array of regulations is to make it difficult for an employer to refuse a request for lactation breaks. How do managers understand this complex regulatory system?

In this chapter, I discuss my research into the legal understandings that managers have of this topic. I give a summary of the key legislation applicable in the UK and discuss how this is applied within the workplace. I also reflect upon my findings and give some suggestions for how to improve the legislative backdrop in which women make decisions about their return to work, breastfeeding and how this process can be better managed by employers.

In the project described here, I asked managers, human resources (HR) staff and strategic leaders in a UK public sector organisation about lactation breaks (Fraser, 2016). This investigation shows a real-world context for decision-making around infant feeding. Managers displayed limited knowledge of the legislation and called for goodwill from all parties to resolve issues, better guidance and perhaps legislation on the topic. There were some hesitancies about allowing a baby to visit the workplace, because of lack of suitable facilities, and health and safety issues. My results indicate that better procedures are needed for the process of returning to work as a new parent, and that lactation breaks should be part of that conversation.

Context

The study discussed in this chapter attends to the context of decisions, rather than focusing on women's choices. Employers' and managers' views have been studied in the US by other researchers (Stratton and Henry, 2011; Bai et al, 2012; Anderson et al, 2015). UK researchers have investigated the context for lactation breaks by asking women about their experiences (see Kosmala-Anderson and Wallace, 2006; Wallace et al, 2008; Gatrell, 2011). My findings are broadly in alignment with their results and further the understandings of contextual issues facing breastfeeding, working mothers. Although mothers in the US work in a very different environment, it seems that the concerns managers have about lactation breaks are similar in both the US and the UK.

The use of a case study is a valuable way to increase the emphasis on context and the circumstances that surround employees contemplating lactation breaks, but all employers are different. My case study employer was a large, family-friendly organisation. Participant group size was small (27 participants), composed of individuals who were likely to be atypically supportive of lactation breaks (because they volunteered to talk about the topic). Moreover, since data collection occurred in 2013, there have been changes in the organisation and it is likely that there would be some differences were the exercise to be repeated now, even if the same methodology was used. These factors impact on the transferability of my findings (Yin, 2012). Conversely, reservations which are expressed by supportive managers are likely to be widespread among all managers, so there are advantages to having selected a supportive sample. Using a case study organisation ensures that research is grounded in a reality. This real-world lens enables a clearer perspective on the issue.

The 27 participants included five men (of whom four were fathers; the remaining one did not disclose his parenting status); 16 were mothers, of whom five had taken lactation breaks. Of the participants, 12 had some experience of lactation breaks and two had personally managed staff who took lactation breaks. The split between managing working-class and middle-class staff was even (seven working class, two of whom were male, and eight middle class, two of whom were male). Class was defined using Office for National Statistics categories (based on information supplied by participants), and equates to the American terms 'blue collar' (working class) and 'white collar' (middle class). Five members of the HR department were also interviewed, as well as seven strategically important personnel, who were identified through a snowball process. I asked participants, including the managing director, who they would consult with queries on the topic. All participants have been given pseudonyms; the organisation has also been anonymised for ethical reasons.

Investigating how law and global policy become relevant and applicable in the lives of individual employees is especially illuminating, as the study crosses law, politics, power relations and personal factors. Employers and managers are stakeholders with considerable power regarding use of working time, which influences the context for lactation breaks. Considering their position is therefore important. My study suggests that managers and employers foresee issues which might make it hard to take lactation breaks. This is despite a combination of law, policy and employer support which is rhetorically in favour of lactation breaks.

The law on lactation breaks

There is no clear statutory provision in the UK granting employees enforceable, unambiguous rights to take lactation breaks. Employers may want employees to return on the same terms and conditions as before they became parents, and may not want to engage with infant feeding issues. However, because of the policy interest in health and wellbeing, and additional issues around women's autonomy, the UK government has produced a range of guidance and legal requirements that employers must be aware of, and compliant with, regarding breastfeeding employees.

The employer is under formal obligation to perform a risk assessment for all lactating staff, to consider any requests for flexible working and to allow unpaid parental leave (The Management of Health and Safety at Work Regulations 1999; The Maternity and Parental Leave etc. Regulations 1999; The Flexible Working Regulations 2014). Night workers who provide appropriate medical evidence are entitled to additional special protection regarding breastfeeding. Employers must avoid indirect sex discrimination, harassment or victimisation, or claims of constructive dismissal arising from lactation breaks (Equality Act 2010). While employers are obliged to provide breastfeeding employees with suitable facilities to rest (normally including the opportunity to lie down), they are not obliged to provide employees with a space to express breast milk (Workplace (Health, Safety and Welfare) Regulations 1992). This subtle distinction means employers are not required to enable lactation breaks, but if they elect not to facilitate them, there is a complex range of legislation to comply with. This is likely to be difficult for employers, and it may be easier to simply provide employees with lactation break facilities.

The Equality Act 2010 defines both direct and indirect discrimination. Direct discrimination is when the victim is treated differently and worse than others because of who they are; indirect discrimination involves the victim being treated the same as others, but it has a different and worse effect upon the victim because of who they are, for example, when a criterion applies to both men and women, but puts women at a disadvantage. Sometimes, indirect discrimination is justified, and not illegal. Discrimination on the grounds of breastfeeding is specifically excluded from being direct discrimination within the workplace under the Equality Act. Previous case law (*Williams v. MOD* [2003] All ER (D) 142) had established the potential for a direct discrimination claim, but this possibility was removed by the Equality Act 2010, so now lactation breaks can only be considered as indirect sex discrimination. This was a deliberate political decision in the light of the fact that the Act describes discrimination regarding breastfeeding as potentially direct discrimination in a non-work context.

European law is also relevant. The Pregnant Workers Directive (92/85/EEC) has been implemented via an array of UK legislation (Workplace (Health, Safety and Welfare) Regulations 1992; Employment Rights Act 1996; Management of Health and Safety at Work Regulations 1999). Article 3 of the Directive contains guidelines for assessing chemical, physical and biological agents and industrial processes which are considered hazardous for breastfeeding workers. Article 4 of the Directive covers risk assessments for breastfeeding workers. There is a non-exhaustive list of hazardous agents, processes and working conditions included in an annex to the Directive. These could include matters such as posture, travel and fatigue.

There are some hints of a 'right to breastfeeding' within human rights law (Hausman, 2004; Kent, 2006). The foundation for a human rights approach to lactation breaks may not have been intended to create such a right when initially drafted, but it could provide the basis for an understanding of breastfeeding as a human right, whether of the mother, the child or both together (Greiner, 1993; Barkhuis, 1994; Bar-Yam, 2003). Lactation breaks are also provided for in International Labour Office Convention 183. However, lack of public awareness and enforceability issues prevent this being widely accessed (Gibbons, 1987). The World Health Organization has also encouraged lactation breaks. Paragraph 45 of the *Global strategy for infant and young child feeding* states:

Employers should ensure maternity entitlements of paid employments of all women in paid employment are met, including breastfeeding breaks or other workplace arrangements – for example, facilities for expressing and storing breastmilk for later feeding by a caregiver – in order to facilitate breast-milk feeding once maternity is over. Trade unions have a direct role in negotiating adequate maternity entitlement and security of employment for women of reproductive age. (WHO and Unicef, 2003: 23)

It is unlikely that many managers will be aware of the full range of legislation and quasi-legislation in relation to the subject of lactation breaks. To refuse a request, an employer would have to be compliant with this range of legislation insofar as it is enforceable against an employer, and this would be hard to do in practice. Many employers will conclude that, given the complexity of the legislation, providing lactation breaks is sensible. In addition to the formal, legal rights, employers may also elect to be guided by non-mandatory government publications (Health and Safety Executive, 2009; ACAS, 2014). These encourage employers to provide staff with lactation breaks but emphasise that the employer is not under an obligation to do so.

Employment contracts are often formed of multiple documents and include a requirement to observe employer policy. Therefore, an employment contract may confer the right to take lactation breaks or specify any conditions associated with such breaks. The right to lactation breaks is not automatically implied in employment contracts under UK law, but there are related rights which are intended to be enforceable within the employment tribunal system. Taken together, this range of legislation is likely to make it difficult for an employer to refuse to accommodate lactation breaks altogether. However, the absence of a clear and unambiguous statutory right for employees, and obligation on employers, to accommodate lactation breaks within the workplace has been identified and criticised by many commentators on the subject (Wood, 2001; Daley and Baker, 2003).

Managers' understanding of and access to the law

Comparisons between lactation breaks and other issues were widespread among participants. Some of these issues included LGBTQ+ and other diversity issues, disability, cycling to work, time off for antenatal appointments, going to the toilet, childcare and eldercare, coffee breaks, going to medical appointments, breaks for health reasons, mobile phone calls being are taken at work, stress-related issues, prayer breaks, and other domestic issues. Storing breast milk in the fridge was compared with a diabetic person storing insulin. A controversial comparison issue was a smoking break – some participants considered whether this was equivalent before rejecting the analogy.

The most common type of law which participants referred to was maternity legislation. Therefore, participants requested advice on how to handle the topic from the HR department, rather than the Health and Safety department. This is intriguing, as UK legislation is primarily focused on health and safety. Participants sometimes mentioned other sources. I asked Ella, an office manager, where she would seek information. She said:

> 'I'd find the [organisation] stuff on the HR website. I'd find the government stuff on the government website. Those are the places you would look for it.' (Ella, Office Manager)

When participants were not aware of the law, they often guessed that the law obliged them to offer employees lactation breaks, but said that they would check. Kaye, a reception manager commented:

> 'I suspect legally that we should allow people to take lactation breaks but then the law is quite progressive and I am not sure so I don't actually know. I would ask HR, they would have a handle on what we're legally supposed to do, or I would Google it.' (Kaye, Reception Manager)

When I prompted managers in my sample, they often considered risk assessments for the woman taking lactation breaks. However, there was some discomfort with the idea of dealing with lactation breaks in health and safety terms. Sophie is an HR officer. I asked her: "Would health and safety be something you would be interested in?" Sophie replied:

> 'Not necessarily, no. I might consult them if we were talking about bringing the baby into work but just ordinarily expressing? I don't think I would talk to them. It wouldn't have sprung to mind. I would say it's an HR thing, but it is a healthy thing.' (Sophie, HR Officer)

I also spoke with Amelia who was the Health and Safety Manager. She felt that the topic was primarily an HR issue. She commented:

'I think the leading of it is more in the HR realm because we don't know who is pregnant and I think it is right that we don't know. It should be dealt with through line management and through HR.' (Amelia, Health and Safety Manager)

Amelia was aware of the health and safety legislative requirements and explained these clearly to me, but she did not feel that lactation breaks fell naturally within her remit.

Managers were also conscious of the need for goodwill, guidance and perhaps legislation. Simon, the Managing Director, comments:

'It's about discussion and negotiation and reasonableness, the minute we lose that and hide behind legislation, we've lost the plot I think.' (Simon, Managing Director)

Simon was therefore keen to deal with the matter in a setting of goodwill from all parties, rather than invoking a rigid statutory framework. He argued against a bureaucratic, legalised approach to some extent by emphasising instead the need for positive relationships and goodwill. Perhaps it is not surprising that Simon would argue for the need for positive relationships and goodwill; he is likely to have both power and a history of successful negotiation in his favour.

However, some managers wanted to have more guidance around the topic. Joan was a catering manager and one of her staff had asked for lactation breaks on her return to work. She commented:

'I don't think there's enough information for managers, or guidance. The one [request for lactation breaks] I had dealt with was quite simple to support, the impact was very small.' (Joan, Catering Manager)

This is intriguing because the organisation had clear policies that Joan could have looked up. But she did not find them accessible and, therefore, as she was able to deal with the matter through goodwill, she did not access the formal guidance. In a situation where there is no goodwill, or where other factors limit the issue, managers recognised the need for legislation and guidance to act as a backstop. Ricky was a manager of a reception desk. He commented:

'Subconsciously and surreptitiously somebody, an unscrupulous manager, could put up multiple barriers to stop someone doing it, but yeah, they could and should and deserve to have the absolute pants sued off them for doing it.' (Ricky, Reception Manager)

This is a very strong statement in support of a legally mandated right to lactation breaks. Ricky is a manager of a reception desk and probably has a different perspective to Simon. It is likely that Ricky experiences less power within the workplace. Therefore, it is also not surprising that Ricky, but not Simon, calls for a legal backstop.

It is also interesting that Ricky develops his opinion in more emphatic terms as he considers the topic. He moves from saying "could" to "could and should", and "deserve". This implies that the more he thinks about it, the more he considers that a legal right, backed up with punitive powers, is required to underpin the obligations upon employers. Ricky's call for the presence of strong punitive measures refers not just to "pants" but to "absolute pants", which are "sued off them". This, particularly the phraseology he has chosen to use, suggests strength of feeling on the topic.

Other managers highlighted that they experienced a lack of legal information on the topic. Sophie was both an HR officer and a former breastfeeding peer supporter. She investigated the legal context prior to our interview, but commented that she was confused:

'We have an online HR employment law. It came up with loads of stuff that I glanced through. It told me every EU country, what the law was, but it didn't answer my specific questions. There were a few bits and pieces I glued together in my head. It wasn't actually in the law specifically, it was just sort of a goodwill gesture. Is that the case? I don't know.' (Sophie, HR Officer)

Sophie has a high level of training on the topic and has taken time to research it but is still uncertain. The absence of a clear legislative steer makes it difficult for her to advise staff who consult her and thus should be seen as a call for clarity on the law on this topic.

Overall, managers understand and access the law by reference to comparative topics and by the range of information they can access. This support was primarily centred in the HR department and internet resources, specifically governmental websites. Health and safety was a factor that managers considered only when prompted. Participants in my sample discussed the law relating to lactation breaks by reference to their wider understandings of similar topics, but would search for information from the internet and the HR department as well. Some mentioned that the information was not easy to find, and members of the HR department were also unclear on both policy and the legislation surrounding it. It seems that situations would often be resolved on an informal basis.

The health and safety manager of the organisation, Amelia, was well informed of the law and could explain the policy within the organisation, but she too felt that it was more appropriate for it to be dealt with through the HR field. Although Amelia acknowledged the existence of variability throughout the organisation, she could provide a concise and accurate precis of the full range of legal rights, and I was impressed with the extent of her knowledge of the subject. The policy that she outlined, which included the provision of rooms to rest and recover, and which she could send me documentation about, was fully congruent with the legal obligations she described. However, she was the only person in my investigations who could reference this policy. The other participants did not know the law or the formal procedures the organisation had in place.

All employing organisations can offer lactation break facilities without any legal framework. However, despite the family-friendly nature of the organisation I studied, there were barriers and restrictions upon staff. Goodwill was foundational for relations on this topic, but participants also wanted guidance. In addition, there was a call for law reform, with some participants calling for an obligation on employers to provide lactation breaks.

Difficulty in accessing law and policy makes it hard for managers to understand and apply the relevant principles about lactation breaks, with consequent potential for inertia. The calls by some study participants for greater guidance, and perhaps legislation on the topic, are directly linked to their level of power within the organisation (Laverack, 2016). There is some evidence of an absence of clearly disseminated guidance and policy. The potential for employees to make a free and empowered choice about lactation breaks is hindered by the realities and constraints experienced in the organisation's context.

Breastfeeding directly at the breast

There was considerable ambiguity among my study participants about bringing children onto the worksite, and the written policy reflected this. A mother experiences many liminal positions within the workplace, moving from pregnancy, to maternity leave, to her return to work (Dowling and Pontin, 2017). Especially during the transition back to being in work, she may wish to bring her baby with her, for instance, during visits while she is on maternity leave or during 'keeping in touch' days. After her return to work, she may wish to bring her baby with her to the workplace for visits. Sometimes, the purpose may be to breastfeed, but her reasons may also relate to childcare or logistics. Often, there will be a mix of reasons, with breastfeeding more significant for younger babies.

However, bringing a baby to work may not be welcomed by employers. They could be concerned about their liability for an infant or the impact on the working culture. Employers may have a variety of strategies and policies which impede the opportunity to bring a baby into the workplace. Thus, a mother may be separated from her baby for institutional reasons, unless she elects to discontinue working. Anne was a middle-class manager who had just returned from maternity leave herself. She explained to me:

> 'This is a place of work, and you could argue that it's not designed for people coming in with babies. Now, there may well be somewhere people can go and change their baby or feed their baby in a quieter place, but I don't know about it, and having just been on maternity leave, you'd think I'd be informed. They stress that you can take breaks to go and feed your baby, but, just from a practical nature, I don't know how that actually happens. Where do you go?' (Anne, Office Manager)

The embodied acts of breastfeeding and expressing breast milk may have different connections and meanings for mothers, and may be interpreted in different ways (Ryan et al, 2013). They could also be perceived differently by managers, co-workers and employees. The baby's experience of receiving breast milk by bottle also deserves close attention (Johnson et al, 2009; Li et al, 2010; Disantis et al, 2011; Dinour et al, 2015). Mothers might not want to express breast milk; they may want to breastfeed directly. Babies might not take bottles; they may want their mother's breast.

Expressing breast milk may not meet the mother's or the baby's needs. My participants acknowledged that the context impacted the mother's autonomy to choose to breastfeed. Sometimes breastfeeding at work might be hard to organise, but expressing milk would be easier for the employer to arrange. Mothers who choose breastfeeding might face obstacles; the realistic, pragmatic issues impede and constrict the availability of options. I asked Jane, an equalities officer, "How do you feel about a mum taking a break during the working day to go and visit her baby and breastfeed?" She considered the issue:

'That's quite a good and forward-thinking idea. Presumably you'd have some sort of nursery facility where the baby is looked after and the mother could go and do that. Yes, I think that's a good idea.' (Jane, Equalities Officer)

However, this doesn't work for all employees. Cleaners often work shifts that don't correspond with nursery hours, and it wouldn't be easy for them to have visits from their baby either:

'Obviously with the job we're doing, you couldn't really have the baby with you because of health and safety.' (Carla, Cleaning Manager)

My participants supported maternal autonomy and this included opportunity to express breastmilk where this was the chosen way to take a lactation break. Although they may have been aware of the arguments concerning the embodied and relational nature of breastfeeding, and that expressing breastmilk is a more technologised option which affects the mother–infant connection, they were not engaged with this argument (Fentiman, 2009; Dykes and Flacking, 2010; Ryan, Team and Alexander, 2013). My participants often construed their role as being a facilitator: to help make mothers' choices to take lactation breaks a reality, considering the context.

Risk assessment on return to work

There is an irony in legally requiring risk assessments to be carried out for women undertaking lactation breaks, as it portrays breastfeeding and lactation breaks as 'risky'. This is echoed by concern for the wellbeing of women taking lactation breaks (but not ascribing risks to weaning). Could this potentially be interpreted as an encouragement to employees to wean their babies? It is at odds with health promotion messaging. Health research has increasingly referenced the risks associated with formula feeding. The risks associated with infant feeding decisions and the terminology with which the potential options are described are emotive. Yet it seems surprising to portray breastfeeding and breast milk expression as a risky activity, particularly given that the alternative is usually the use of infant formula, for which no risk assessment is performed. It is also odd to be concerned for employees because they are breastfeeding, given the value of breastfeeding for women's health. Early weaning has implications for maternal and infant health (Bernshaw, 2009; Quigley, 2013; Victora et al, 2016).

Performing risk assessments for women who are breastfeeding or expressing breast milk implies that there are risks associated with lactation, although continuing to breastfeed is not a risk to health. Ceasing to breastfeed and using infant formula could be seen as increasing the risk to both mother's and baby's health (Arneil, 2000; Wallace et al, 2011). So it is bizarre that the law requires a risk assessment for the breastfeeding/expressing mother, without considering the risks for mothers who return to work having weaned to formula. This is a legal signal which implies that formula feeding is less risky than breastfeeding – a complete contradiction to the health messaging.

All new parents potentially encounter issues such as stress, fatigue, role adjustment issues and depression. Returning to work after maternity, paternity or adoption leave is a potentially fraught time (Foli et al, 2015; Giallo and Cooklin, 2015). All parents face this, so perhaps a risk assessment is always appropriate on return to work. One item of that assessment might be the risk of early weaning, which would then open discussion about lactation breaks. This would also address the feature of my study, in which conversations about lactation breaks did not appear to be happening on a routine basis. Interestingly, participants were willing to discuss the topic and look for ways to support lactation breaks, when they became aware of it as a factor. A clear legislative right to take lactation breaks during working time would be useful in providing employers with guidance. There are already so many complex legal rights that it is hard to refuse lactation breaks, but the legislative backdrop is confusing for managers. This lack of clarity was regarded as unhelpful by participants in this study.

Debates about lactation breaks

Some of the feminist positions surrounding lactation breaks, and the debate engendered, have been summarised by other writers (Van Esterik, 1989; Galtry, 2000; McCarter-Spaulding, 2008; Lee, 2012). By addressing the context, I am incorporating both public health and autonomy-based advocacy in relation to the topic. My research attempts to synthesise different feminist positions by respecting choice and, simultaneously, health and wellbeing issues. It also addresses criticisms about overzealous promotion of breastfeeding and autonomy. This research aims to address structural supports and limitations around lactation breaks, while respecting maternal autonomy and resisting shame. Some of the negative guilt feelings can be conceptualised as including anger and frustration at the limitations new mothers experience in their lived context (Labbok, 2008; Forster and McLachlan, 2010; Ryan et al, 2011). Addressing issues of the circumstances, information, support and options that mothers experience may therefore be a liberating, feminist experience for new mothers.

Requiring risk assessments for all new parents who are combining working with a new baby, which includes an assessment of the risk of early weaning, as well as fatigue, depression and so on, is a way to provide an approach which unites all new parents and does not discriminate against a single group. It would help overcome the 'mummy wars', while still respecting public health issues concerning the importance of breastfeeding (Bernshaw, 2009). By examining a range of postnatal risks and compiling a set of strategies to address them in the workplace, the risks associated with early weaning might be perceived in an appropriate context. Highlighting breastfeeding as potentially risky would be contextualised by examining the risk of a mother ceasing to breastfeed. The range of arguments in relation to 'why take lactation breaks?' may be better communicated to a range of employees and managers when the risks of early weaning are addressed.

A risk assessment for all new parents would also enable managers to formalise some of the concerns and desire to support their staff. The caring attitude of my participants towards their postnatal employees, which included all mothers whether they desired to take lactation breaks or not, was strongly supported within my data. A risk assessment for all new parents would enable greater discussions to be had on a range of factors about how the postnatal status and working patterns might coexist, and enable positive solutions to be found which respect the autonomy of the new parent and the working conditions of the employer.

Conclusion

While lactation breaks continue to be a vexed topic with contextual barriers, even within supportive organisations such as this case study organisation, there will continue to be a need for alternative strategies to enable mothers to breastfeed their babies. These supportive working practices, such as the availability of paid maternity leave and flexible or part-time options on the return to work, remain important for women. This discussion will therefore be useful for both policy makers and practitioners working with mothers returning to work and assessing their options. As the study discussed here demonstrates, even within supportive environments, lactation breaks remain a contested area.

.

References

Advisory, Conciliation, and Arbitration Service (2014) *Accommodating breastfeeding employees in the workplace*, www.acas.org.uk/media/pdf/j/k/Acas_guide_on_accommodating_breastfeeding_in_the_workplace_(JANUARY2014).pdf

Anderson, J., Kuehl, R. A., Drury, S. A., Tschetter, L., Schwaegerl, M., Hildreth, M., Bachman, C., Gullickson, H., Yoder, J. and Lamp, J. (2015) 'Policies aren't enough: the importance of interpersonal communication about workplace breastfeeding support', *Journal of Human Lactation,* 31(2): 260–66.

Arneil, B. (2000) 'The politics of the breast', *Canadian Journal of Women and the Law*, 12(2): 345–70.

Bai, Y. K., Wunderlich, S. M. and Weinstock, M. (2012) 'Employers' readiness for the mother-friendly workplace: an elicitation study', *Maternal and Child Nutrition*, (8)4: 483–91.

Barkhuis, S. S. (1994) 'Breast-feeding and the law', *Texas Journal of Women and the Law*, (3): 417–46.

Bar-Yam, N. B. (2003) 'Breastfeeding and human rights: is there a right to breastfeed?', *Journal of Human Lactation,* 19(4): 357–61.

Bernshaw, N. J. (2009) 'Breastfeeding should be expressed as the norm', *Journal of Human Lactation*, 25(1): 10.

Daley, B. and Baker, S. (2003) 'A right to breastfeed?', *Employment Law Journal*, 46: 5–6.

Dinour, L. M., Pope, G. A. and Bai, Y. K. (2015) 'Breast milk pumping beliefs, supports, and barriers on a university campus', *Journal of Human Lactation*, 31(1): 156–65.

Disantis, K. I., Collins, B. N., Fisher, J. O. and Davey, A. (2011) 'Do infants fed directly from the breast have improved appetite regulation and slower growth during early childhood compared with infants fed from a bottle?', *The International Journal of Behavioral Nutrition and Physical Activity*, 8: 89.

Dowling, S. and Pontin, D. 2017, 'Using liminality to understand mothers' experiences of long-term breastfeeding: "Betwixt and between", and "matter out of place",' *Health*, 21(1): 57–75.

Dykes, F. and Flacking, R. (2010) 'Encouraging breastfeeding: a relational perspective', *Early Human Development*, 86(11): 733–6.Fentiman, L. C. (2009) 'Marketing mothers' milk: the commodification of breastfeeding and the new markets in human milk and infant formula', *Nevada Law Review*, 10 (1): 29–81.

Foli, K. J., Lim, E. and Sands, L. P. (2015) 'Comparison of relative and non-relative adoptive parent health status', *Western Journal of Nursing Research*, 37(3): 320–41.

Forster, D. A. and McLachlan, H. L. (2010) 'Women's views and experiences of breast feeding: positive, negative or just good for the baby?', *Midwifery*, 26(1): 116–25.

Fraser, M. A. (2016) 'Managers' perspectives of lactation breaks: the context of infant feeding decisions among staff in one public sector organisation' [unpublished doctoral dissertation], Bristol: University of the West of England.

Galtry, J. (2000) 'Extending the "bright line": feminism, breastfeed and the workplace in the United States', *Gender and Society*, 14: 295–317.

Gatrell, C. (2011) 'Managing the maternal body: a comprehensive review and transdisciplinary analysis', *International Journal of Management Reviews*, 13(1): 97–112.

Giallo, R. and Cooklin, A. (2015) 'Guest editorial: special issue on parent mental health', *Clinical Psychologist*, 19(1): 1–2.

Gibbons, G. (1987) 'Legislation, women, and breastfeeding', *MCH News PAC*, 2(4): 5–11.

Greiner, T. (1993) 'Breastfeeding and maternal employment: another perspective', *Journal of Human Lactation,* 9(4): 214–15.

Hausman, B. L. (2004) 'The feminist politics of breastfeeding', *Australian Feminist Studies*, 19(45): 273–85.

Health and Safety Executive (2009) 'A guide for new and expectant mothers who work', www.hse.gov.uk/pubns/indg373.pdf

International Labour Organization, C183 Maternity Protection Convention, 2000 (No 183), www.ilo.org

Johnson, S., Williamson, I., Lyttle, S. and Leeming, D. (2009) 'Expressing yourself: a feminist analysis of talk around expressing breast milk', *Social Science and Medicine*, 69(6): 900–907.

Kent, G. (2006) 'Child feeding and human rights', *International Breastfeeding Journal*, 1: 27.

Kosmala-Anderson, J. and Wallace, L. M. (2006) 'Breastfeeding works: the role of employers in supporting women who wish to breastfeed and work in four organizations in England', *Journal of Public Health*, 28: 183–91.

Labbok, M. (2008) 'Exploration of guilt among mothers who do not breastfeed: the physician's role', *Journal of Human Lactation*, 24(1): 80–84.

Laverack, G. (2016) *Public health: Power, empowerment and professional practice*, (3rd edn), London: Palgrave.

Lee, R. (2012) 'Breastfeeding and constraints on mother's agency', *Motherhood Activism, Advocacy, Agency*, (3)2: 93–102.

Li, R., Fein, S. B. and Grummer-Strawn, L. M. (2010), 'Do infants fed from bottles lack self-regulation of milk intake compared with directly breastfed infants?', *Pediatrics*, 125(6): 1386–93.

McCarter-Spaulding, D. (2008) 'Is breastfeeding fair? Tensions in feminist perspectives on breastfeeding and the family', *Journal of Human Lactation*, 24(20): 206–12.

Quigley, M. A. (2013) 'Breast feeding, causal effects and inequalities', *Archives of Disease in Childhood*, 98(9): 654–5.

Ryan, K., Todres, L. and Alexander, J. (2011) 'Calling, permission, and fulfillment: the interembodied experience of breastfeeding', *Qualitative Health Research*, 21(6): 731–42.

Ryan, K., Team, V. and Alexander, J. (2013) 'Expressionists of the twenty-first century: the commodification and commercialization of expressed breast milk', *Medical Anthropology*, 32(5): 467–86.Stratton, J. and Henry, B. W. (2011) 'What employers and health care providers can do to support breastfeeding in the workplace: aiming to match positive attitudes with action', *Infant, Child, and Adolescent Nutrition*, 3(5): 300–307.

Van Esterik, P. (1989) *Motherpower and infant feeding*, London: Zed Books.

Victora, C. G., Bahl, R., Barros, A.J.D., França, G.V.A., Horton, S., Krasevec, J., Murch, S., Sankar, M. J., Walker, N. and Rollins, N. C., on behalf of The Lancet Breastfeeding Series Group (2016), 'Breastfeeding in the 21st century: epidemiology, mechanisms, and lifelong effect', *Lancet*, 387(10017): 475–90.

Wallace, L.J.E. and Taylor, E. N. (2011) 'Potential risks of "risk" language in breastfeeding advocacy', *Women and Health*, 51(4): 299–320.

Wallace, L., Kosmala-Anderson, J., Mills, S., Law, S., Skinner, D., Bayley, J. and Baum, A. (2008) 'Mutually exclusive? A United Kingdom survey of women's experiences of breastfeeding and working', *MIDIRS Midwifery Digest*, 18(1): 99–103.

Wood, K. (2001) *Maternity and parental rights: A practical guide*, London: The Stationery Office.

World Health Organization and Unicef (2003) *Global strategy for infant and young child feeding*, Geneva: WHO.

Yin, R. K. (2012) *Applications of case study research*, Los Angeles, CA: Sage.

TEN

Making breastfeeding social: the role of brelfies in breastfeeding's burgeoning publics

Fiona Giles

Introduction

This chapter looks at the online circulation of breastfeeding selfies –
or brelfies – and asks what their benefits might be in terms of making
breastfeeding easier. It looks at brelfies as social media activism, drawing
attention to embodied mothering, and upending assumptions about
the solitary nature of maternity. It argues that brelfies provide a means
through which breastfeeding can emerge from its existing practical,
conceptual and imaginary confines, by communicating images of
breastfeeding to an almost limitless audience.

Not only have brelfies attracted extensive media coverage, raising
awareness about breastfeeding in the community, the images also
provide a unique form of communication between breastfeeding
mothers and their friends, families and children, as mothers see
themselves in the act of taking their own photos. By considering the
implications of increased images of women breastfeeding in public –
as well as the increased circulation of images of women breastfeeding
generally – this chapter argues that brelfies invite us to reconceptualise
breastfeeding in public as breastfeeding in social contexts more broadly:
in short, to reimagine breastfeeding in relation to its many publics.

To date, the challenges of breastfeeding in public have been conceived
against the norm of breastfeeding in private. The two spaces are
regarded as distinct, with private breastfeeding referring to the mother
breastfeeding her child in her home, either alone or with her family.
Breastfeeding in public has referred to a contrasting experience, when
a mother breastfeeds anywhere outside this space. Yet breastfeeding at
home may also take place in social if not public contexts, with family,
friends or other visitors present, and the mother may feel obliged to

withdraw into a more private space. Private breastfeeding is therefore solitary, the only human company being the feeding child.

Breastfeeding in public may also require the mother to find spaces that accommodate solitude, so that so-called 'breastfeeding in public' takes place in a toilet cubicle, parents' room, or a secluded corner of a shopping centre or car park. Is a breastfeeding mother sitting in her car while parked on the street engaged in public or private breastfeeding? If she has retreated to a toilet cubicle, has she achieved privacy, or merely a moment of solitude in a public space?

Although a more useful distinction might be made between solitary and social breastfeeding, it is important to recognise that breastfeeding is an inherently social activity, because the mother is engaged in an act of embodied communication with her child. The two individuals (or three in the case of twins or older nursing siblings) are not only nursing and being nursed, they are keeping each other company. Breastfeeding signifies the origins of sociality for our species, our capacity for empathy, and is one of our most vital forms of affective and biochemical interaction (Yalom, 1997; Angiers, 1999; Hrdy, 1999). Researchers administering oxytocin to adults with autism know that this chemical, abundant during lactation, significantly improves social responsiveness (Yatawara et al, 2016). The psychological coming-into-being of the infant through exchanging its gaze with its mother, or seeing its image reflected in her eye, is also a bringing-into-sociality of the subject (Lacan, 2001 [1949]). Additionally, the exchange of sustenance and antibodies ushers the child into the microbial sociality underpinning our immune function (Gribble, 2005; Hird, 2007).

In addition to the undeniable sociality of breastfeeding, the private/ public binary reinforces the fictional division between private and public personae, which many scholars have critiqued as delusory (Plummer, 2003). It could be argued that the early feminist slogan 'the personal is political' announced its end (Hanisch, 1970). Particularly when engaged in maternal labour, maintaining a clear-cut boundary between private and public, as well as self and other, is simply untenable. As Ruddick (1989) argues, motherwork entails the preservation, defence and training of children, each performed through interdependence. Maternal relationality ushers young subjects into a socio-moral order that is itself profoundly relational (Hamington, 2004; Held, 2006). Similar arguments are made in feminist critiques of neoliberal conceptions of selfhood, revealing how the ideal of the individual subject upon which this ideology relies, bears little resemblance to the inescapable interdependence of all humans (Manne, 2005; Stephens, 2012; Hamilton, 2017). By shifting our attention to the social dimensions of mothering, we may bypass the divisiveness that pits women's allegedly private concerns against the legitimated, masculinised public concerns of the self-reliant wage-earner, who brackets out his or her parenting identity for times of public engagement, or remains childless.

For all these reasons, I propose that breastfeeding needs to be acknowledged as a social behaviour, deserving more comprehensive appreciation of its complex webs of intersubjectivity. By doing so, breastfeeding may be accommodated as a layer of sociality integral to, or at least continuous with, sociality's many other manifestations. This is not merely to support mothers to breastfeed confidently in spaces beyond their homes; it is also to invite them into shared social spaces: at the table, at work, and in the many other spaces of conviviality. Conceiving of breastfeeding as social acknowledges how it underpins hospitality, the welcoming of another into a space of generosity and sharing (Hamington, 2004; Held, 2006; Lee, 2016), and literally enacts commensal relations where humans share sustenance for mutual benefit (Van Esterik, 2015). To deny breastfeeding its rightful place within the social not only deprives mothers and babies of company, it also depletes social gatherings of their lifeblood.

Social media activism and the role of the image

The role of brelfies in making breastfeeding social happens on at least two planes. First, it enables the image of the mother breastfeeding, wherever this takes place, to reach a wider public, in the sense of a public as an audience. In this sense, it socialises the image itself: whether that be to a group of friends on a Facebook page, to a broader audience subscribing to an Instagram account or via Twitter hashtags and news media. Second, through the communicative gesture of a mother taking a photo of herself and her child nursing, she invites that audience to join her, and she extends the hospitality inherent in the act of nursing to the hospitality of inviting company into her enchanted circle. Her brelfie image says, 'Here I am with my child, and I am warmly inviting you to join me in this space.' Her point is not to reinscribe the public/private binary, but to dismantle the solitary/social one.

Nevertheless, it is important to acknowledge that expanding the breastfeeding imaginary is insufficient for achieving social change on its own. A recent study of online comments responding to images of military women breastfeeding showed how, even as media framing became more positive between 2012 and 2015, negative attitudes persisted within the broader community (Midberry, 2017). Attitude change can take decades; and while significant progress has been made in expanding the diversity of and audience for breastfeeding images since the 1990s, anger is still being expressed by some concerning what they see as breaches of breastfeeding protocols. In addition to changing attitudes, mothers also need structural reform and material support beyond the symbolic for their free and open practice of maternal labour (Hausman, 2003, 2012; Knaak, 2005; Smyth, 2009). Accommodating women's breastfeeding needs at work, providing adequate parental leave, and designing spaces catering to the needs of mothers and babies, both within and beyond domestic settings, all contribute to making breastfeeding more feasible.

Yet structural reforms are also insufficient. Legislation in many countries now protects women's right to breastfeed in public; and in Scotland, a fine of up to £2,500 may be imposed for preventing breastfeeding of a child up to two years of age in any location (Scotland Act, 2005). Yet in France, where it is also legal to breastfeed in public, breastfeeding rates are among the lowest in the West, and women are rarely seen breastfeeding outside the home (Komodiki, 2014). Normalisation may only be achieved if mothers can represent themselves as active agents of the maternal work of breastfeeding, and active agents of their own image-making and distribution. Expanding the breastfeeding imaginary is a vital adjunct to achieving, as well as representing, this change (Britton, 2009).

Media campaigns have long seen attitudinal change and awareness-raising as their primary objectives (Wakefield, 2010; Freeman et al, 2015). But this is insufficient and may have unintended consequences. A report from of a poll carried out in England in 2015 showed that while 72% of people surveyed thought women should feel comfortable breastfeeding in public, 60% of mothers said they try to hide what they're doing (Public Health England, 2015). While media reports of public breastfeeding controversies can inspire nurse-ins and publicise women's rights, they may also give the impression that harassment is more common than is the case. It is therefore important for part of this attitudinal change to be driven by mothers themselves, instilling confidence in their entitlement and ability to breastfeed in public by posting images as they do so (Bandura, 1982).

The circulation of images is also vital to laying the groundwork for acceptance. As Penny writes in *Unspeakable things*, 'Throughout human history, the most important political battles have been fought on the territory of the imagination, and what stories we allow ourselves to tell depend on what we can imagine' (Penny, 2014: 1). Similarly, Bartlett states in *Breastwork*, 'Valuing of breastfeeding life must take place at the level of thinking and representation in order to make the link between cultural representation and practice' (Bartlett, 2005: 186). It is not only being seen that counts. It is also necessary for the mother to announce herself – and to produce her image – as worthy of spectatorship. Tugwell's analysis of Catherine Opie's *Self-Portrait/ Nursing* (2004) shows that it is vital to represent the mother as 'a desiring social subject' on the occasion of breastfeeding. As Tugwell writes: 'to explore the female imaginary is to imagine the unimaginable, a way of opening a space for exploration and expression' (2013: 8). No less than the recognition of cultures' 'debt to the maternal' more broadly, and 'the continuous connection to the mother in psychic life' are at stake in making breastfeeding visible (2013: 48).

The advent of the brelfie

The term brelfie, to describe a selfie posted by a mother while breastfeeding, was coined in December 2014, when actress Alyssa Milano posted a selfie while feeding her three-month-old daughter Elizabella Dylan on Instagram. Milano received criticism for her posting, which in turn instigated support, and she then set up the hashtag 'brelfie', although the original posting and news coverage referred to the photo as a 'breastfeeding selfie' (Gibbs Vengrow, nd; Milano, 2014). Following Milano's hashtag, the first publicly reported use of the term brelfie to mean a breastfeeding selfie was in May 2015, linking it explicitly to its communicative role as the 'posting of intimate shots online' (Open Macmillan Dictionary). The brelfie has therefore had from the start an element of political protest. Milano's brelfie was immediately framed politically, as either promoting breastfeeding in public or transgressing breastfeeding protocol (O'Connor, 2015). Additionally, the term's reference to posting images online – publicising a contested site of intimate conduct – is possibly one of the most vivid examples of visual protest since bra-burning in the 1960s.

Just prior to this time, in March 2015, a protest action of posting breastfeeding selfies on Facebook followed the site's decision to take down photos of a woman breastfeeding, on the grounds that nipples are indecent (White, 2014). In the same month, after campaigning by mothers since 2008, Facebook adjusted its take-down policy to allow breastfeeding selfies. In its press release Facebook states: 'we always allow photos of women actively engaged in breast-feeding or showing breasts with post-mastectomy scarring' (Vnuk, 2015). While this was a breakthrough in the freedom of expression for nursing mothers, Facebook's use of the rhetoric of medicalisation laid bare its ambivalence about images of breastfeeding. Instead of simply acknowledging women's right to represent themselves breastfeeding, Facebook conflated breastfeeding images with images of post-surgical scarring. Lactation and breast cancer were rendered equivalently pathological, disavowing breastfeeding as perfectly normal behaviour sanctioned by the state.

Brelfie hashtags quickly proliferated internationally. The term brelfie was covered widely in the media, and, despite naysayers, over 25% of new mothers had posted or intended to post brelfies in early 2015 (Waterlow, 2015). Throughout 2016 the phenomenon continued to attract numerous media reports of its popularity (Kirwan-Taylor, 2016). Images of celebrities breastfeeding also abounded, and − as with Milano's tabloid appeal − provided more media coverage to the cause than non-celebrity women might have achieved. While many of these photos were taken by others, their popularity and careful staging indicates the importance to the personal and professional identities of these women of not only breastfeeding, but being seen to breastfeed in public. The circumstances within which women were depicted also varied widely; models, musicians and actresses were shown breastfeeding in the workplace, as well as at leisure in outdoor locations. Twitter hashtags, Facebook groups and Instagram accounts included #brelfie, #breastfeedingselfie, #normalizebreasteeding, #breastmilk, #breastisbest and #whereareyoubreastfeedingtoday.

Throughout the past decade, breastfeeding portraiture was showcased by photographers such as Tara Ruby and Ivette Ivens, and promoted by outlets such as the Cosmo series in 2016, Breastfeeding in Real Life, and the Honest Body Project.[1] These portray women breastfeeding in a variety of places and situations, and are commercial, artistic and political projects. Considering that 10 years ago it was rare to see images of breastfeeding outside of fine art contexts, churches or advocacy material, these represent a significant advance in the acceptance of breastfeeding as an activity with everyday aesthetic value (Saito, 2007). The breastfeeding websites also show these images are not merely for the personal record; many have activist objectives: to show what breastfeeding can look like, to reveal the diversity of mothers' bodies and breastfeeding relationships, to illustrate how breastfeeding can be practised in a variety of contexts, and to prove that its everyday

---

[1] See www.parents.com/baby/all-about-babies/alyssa-milanos-breastfeeding-selfie-has-nursing-moms-fired-up/, www.ivetteivens.com/, http://publicbreastfeedingawarenessproject.com/, http://thehonestbodyproject.com/?tag=breastfeeding

aesthetics can be enjoyed by a wide audience. The rise of brelfies took place within this increasingly supportive context of image-making.

The politics of brelfies

With over 310 million Twitter subscribers, 150 million Instagram accounts, and 1.65 billion active users on Facebook, the political potential of social media is well established. In their article 'Breastfeeding selfies and the performance of motherhood', Boon and Pentney (2015) list four values of breastfeeding selfies. First, their pedagogical role helps other mothers see breastfeeding from the point of view of the breastfeeding mother. This enables women to see the range of positions and infant feeding behaviours that are normal, rather than viewing breastfeeding diagrams or photographs taken from the viewer's perspective. It also enables women to imagine themselves breastfeeding, rather than being situated as onlookers. Second, brelfies perform a political function in critiquing the patriarchal ownership of the breast, by showing the baby's behaviour in relation to the breast while feeding. The images claim maternal authority by asserting the agency of the mother to post the photograph. As opposed to feeding in public because her child needs feeding, and seeking to make this occasion less visible, the photographs represent the mothers' decision to feed as an act of self-determination wherever she might happen to be. Third, by drawing attention to realistic images of female embodiment, the maternal body becomes better understood and more openly accepted, in contrast to its concealment or idealisation. Finally, the brelfie shifts attention from face to breast, which, in looming large in relation to the baby, represents both maternal generosity and maternal power and authority. As Boon and Pentney explain, 'This dual agency, by its very nature, disrupts traditional philosophical understandings of the autonomous subject' (2015: 1764).

Other breastfeeding scholars have argued that acknowledging the breastfeeding mother's dual agency and interdependence has a queering effect, showing how assumptions concerning the borders of individual subjectivity are inadequate to both understanding breastfeeding in particular, and the maternal subject more broadly (Giles, 2004; Hausman, 2004; Hird, 2007; Campo, 2010). By extension, public policy based on the needs of individuals as understood within neoliberalism is unlikely to be helpful, since it fails to acknowledge mothers' intersubjectivity, particularly while breastfeeding. What Stephens has described as the post-maternal leanings of neoliberalism further erases the maternal subject, whether conceived of as interdependent or otherwise; she speaks of 'the out-sourced self' in describing how neoliberal policy affects mothers' experiences of maternal labour (Stephens, 2015).

A series of breastfeeding images – #thisishowwecoverup – explicitly disrupts this ideal of the neatly separable individual subject, raising the question: where or who is the self that is being asked to 'cover up' when breastfeeding in public? The most striking of these images shows a woman in a cafe under a sign, which reads: 'If you need to breastfeed … please cover yourself. Thank you.' The mother's response to this instruction is to place her baby's blanket over her own head while leaving her breastfeeding baby and her own upper body clearly visible. The image inspired other women to post brelfies using this hashtag, with their faces covered or disguised. These include a woman breastfeeding while wearing a mask of the *Star Wars* character Darth Vader. The images provide a witty riposte to injunctions for veiling, drawing attention to the pointlessness of the covering edict if the mother's face may be seen: despite covering her baby, the mother is nevertheless 'outed' as a public breastfeeder, which even if performed according to the standards of discretion imposed by some, will nevertheless continue to draw condemnation from others. As Bueskens (2015) has insightfully noted, restrictions on breastfeeding in public are a form of veiling in the West.

In addition to the expansion of diverse images and the multiple perspectives brelfies offer, they also provide an opportunity for women to determine how they would like to be seen, in what platforms and by whom. Whether shot while at home or outside, veiled or naked, they make their mothering public – publicised and published. Posting a brelfie is an act of self-determination that may have radical effects on how that woman imagines herself in her role as both mother and citizen.

The hashtag #thisishowwecoverup draws attention to the range of uncertainties that breastfeeding-in-public protocols are based on: is it the mother's breast, or her identity signified by her face, that is considered out of place? And what of the face of the baby when the mother observes the edict to cover her nursing? Is it, too, an object out of place when suckling at the breast? As Douglas wrote in Purity and danger (2002 [1966]), definitions of culture rest on excluding unacceptable elements of human conduct and embodiment. These are designated not only as intrinsically disorderly or dangerous, but as 'matter out of place' (2002 [1966]: 36). Douglas writes that this fear, which 'inhibits reason', was 'inexplicably confused with defilement and hygiene' (p 1). In turn, the focus on ideals of hygiene leads her to the conclusion 'that some pollutions are used as social analogies for expressing a general view of the social order' (p 3). If an important part of maternal care, as Ruddick defines it, is bringing the child into this social order (through 'training'), how does banishment from view of the mother's fundamental role to feed her offspring affect her own and her child's sense of belonging? How does it affect her moral authority to visibly enact motherwork? A mother who erases her body, the body of her breastfeeding child, her own or her child's face, accepts the same injunction: to erase the significance of maternity at large.

Brelfies as consciousness-raising

Despite their popularity among breastfeeding women, to what extent might brelfies change attitudes more generally? As Boon and Pentney ask, 'Can this form of "gentle" resistance be understood by viewers, or does it collapse into a further reification of the maternal ideal?' (2015: 1765). One answer is provided in an image which makes the brelfie-taker's motivations explicit. It depicts a woman tandem breastfeeding her children on her bed, with superscript that reads as follows: 'I don't share my breastfeeding photos because I think they will change the minds of those who think differently. I share my breastfeeding photos to show the people who already think like me that they are not alone'.

In her book *Mommyblogs*, Friedman (2003) argues that sharing self-representations of maternal experiences, whether in speech, writing, video or photographs, has an important consciousness-raising function. As Friedman (2003) and Kenny (2016) also argue in relation to mommyblogging, there are clear parallels between the 1960s and '70s phenomenon of women's coming to awareness of their collective oppression, and the current coming to awareness of the collective oppression of mothering – in this case raising awareness about breastfeeding.

In addition to communicating normality, having a baby in the photo can also detract from women's anxieties about body image, enabling women to share diverse body types in a supportive environment. As Tiidenberg and Cruz argue in relation to sharing sexually explicit selfies, 'The body-positive atmosphere comes about through the spiral of sharing and learning new ways of looking. It encourages people to put their body out there by soothing their pre-emptive worries about whether it is good enough to be publicly exhibited' (Tiidenberg and Cruz, 2015: 86).

Brelfies therefore fulfil important functions that open out the breastfeeding experience for mothers, communicating the diversity of women's bodies, babies' breastfeeding styles and the places that breastfeeding occurs, assisting mothers in successfully breastfeeding by seeing how breastfeeding works from the perspective of the mother and child, by permitting their breastfeeding to be visible, by allowing the experience to be shared socially, and by demonstrating the importance of breastfeeding to a fuller appreciation of maternal (inter)subjectivity.

The images also resist reification because although many are conservative, in the sense that they depict mostly genteel occasions with babies encircled in their mothers' arms, there are also many that depart from these norms, including breastfeeding children old enough to stand, and mothers in a multitude of spaces, including tourist resorts, public transport, even the London Eye. One image shows a woman doing a handstand with her child lying on the grass beneath her while breastfeeding (Huffington Post, 2013). Even when the traditional hold is used, the majority of the images show the mother looking at the camera, acknowledging her audience, and inviting the return of its gaze, rather than being absorbed demurely, or hiding, within the exclusive view of her baby. The direction of the mother's gaze is of particular importance in understanding the radical potential of brelfies. Not only does the selfie as a genre collapse the object and subject, since they are one and the same (as *I* take a photograph of my self), it also enables a self-fashioning that can disrupt dominant discourses.

From breastfeeding in public to breastfeedings' publics

For the first time, brelfies enable the subjectivity of the breastfeeding mother to be directly communicated as a form of display, specifically for an audience, whether that be a performance for Facebook friends or an unknown public. In the process, she becomes a self-determined performer of her breastfeeding practice and invokes, specifically, an audience. By extension, brelfies enable a shift in our conceptualisation of breastfeeding in public to the idea of breastfeeding having many publics. By taking and posting brelfies, breastfeeding mothers acknowledge their performativity, and take control of the spectacle of breastfeeding to non–breastfeeding others. Rather than seek invisibility of the kinds women have traditionally used to avoid inciting antisocial responses, they stake a claim to their rights as public maternal citizens, and resist the injunction to bear responsibility for the feelings of antagonistic strangers.

This is not to deny that breastfeeding in public, as it is currently understood and studied, remains a critical area of advocacy for the success of breastfeeding generally. As Dowling et al write:

for women to be successful at breastfeeding, they have to be able to breastfeed in public ... To be successful breastfeeders, women must feed their babies when they are hungry – wherever they are ... [and] Where breastfeeding in public is more acceptable, initiation and duration rates appear to be higher. (Dowling et al, 2012: 250)

Yet this conceptualisation of breastfeeding in public need not limit the way women breastfeed in relation to others who are also familial or social, and which social interactions around breastfeeding might (or might not) take place publicly yet within private domains, that is, socially. At the same time, there are enclosed spaces that women can retreat to while breastfeeding in public, which puts them at risk precisely because they are concealed and rendered vulnerable through the absence of familiar company.

Viewing breastfeeding in public as distinct from domestic, home-based breastfeeding not only rests on the binary of private vs public, which is collapsed by social media, it also fails to acknowledge that we have myriad publics, some of which we may interact with in so-called private domains. This leads to counterproductive efforts to make breastfeeding in public safer by providing secluded spaces to breastfeed outside the home. For example, in San Luis Obispo in California, a trial of 'nursing nooks' was established to offer women a 'safe space' in which to breastfeed (Doshier, 2015). While appearing to be supportive of breastfeeding, these are part of an apparatus of lactational regulation. As Lane argues, two arguments are put forward in support of women's right to breastfeed in public: that it is the best source of nutrition for babies, and that women can be supported to breastfeed discreetly. Both rationales use conservative reasoning to 'discipline women and maintain public space-as-usual' (Lane, 2014: 195). She writes:

Although breastfeeding women do nurse in public space with much success, these women discuss and perform the act of breastfeeding in an almost prescriptive manner ... In short, to be considered a good mother, women, if they do nurse their children, must perform breastfeeding a specific way – that is, in a manner that does not have any ostensible (or, worse yet, flagrant) overlap with the performance of sexuality (2014: 207)

The critical element regarding breastfeeding protocols in any space is to do with social relations, whether these are with strangers in a shopping mall or family members over dinner at home, or even child healthcare nurses in a waiting room, whom one researcher observed turning away to offer breastfeeding patients 'privacy' (Mahon-Daly and Andrews, 2002). In looking at images of women breastfeeding outside the home, most women are breastfeeding alone, with their child. Being outside doesn't guarantee company. There are very few images of women breastfeeding socially or at the shared table. It is not surprising they sometimes feel vulnerable.

Conclusion: making breastfeeding social

The company of others is a good thing most of the time, while allowing for periods of solitude. Recognising that we live and eat while engaging with others, it makes sense to welcome breastfeeding into our broader social experience. Moving from the concept of a spatial or civic public into which mothers and children might occasionally venture, to a concept of publics with which mothers and children engage in a myriad of circumstances and spaces, would assist in accommodating the needs of mothers without condemning them to seclusion. When mother and child are completely alone in private, then breastfeeding is not public, though it could be said that they are, at any time, a public of their own making.

As Mahon-Daly and Andrews have shown, breastfeeding currently occurs within a liminal space, and the time of nursing also represents a period of liminality in the life of the mother as citizen (2002; see also Chapter Three in this volume). This requires a self-effacement, so that the nursing mother becomes a spectral presence, shadowy and insignificant, yet threatening nonetheless. By thinking of breastfeeding as taking place within liminal spaces and times, we can move away from the public/private dichotomy and ask how that sense of liminality could be mitigated. For example, to what extent can the liminal maintain its status once it becomes social? Brelfies offer a conceptual trajectory, then, from breastfeeding in public to social breastfeeding, wherever it is performed. Brelfies demonstrate a shift from seeking permission to breastfeed when others are present to celebrating breastfeeding as a socially integrated activity, by representing it as it occurs, and when 'babies ... are hungry – wherever they are' (Dowling et al, 2012: 250). As Shaw and McBride-Henry write, 'To be absorbed and involved in an activity (such as breastfeeding), one needs to feel thoroughly at home in the world, and at home in and with one's body as it is lived and as others see it' (2010: 202). This means planning spaces to foster conviviality more broadly. It also means encouraging women to represent themselves 'with one's body as it is lived'.

The circulation of diverse images of women breastfeeding, taken by breastfeeding women, increases the world's homeliness. The generosity extended through the brelfie gesture also reinscribes breastfeeding as an act of hospitality, an occasion for welcoming company. Hospitality fosters mutuality and a willingness to accommodate needs, including those of strangers, reinforcing our 'intercorporeal existence' (Shaw, 2004: 287). When the image of breastfeeding is communicated by the mother herself, breastfeeding invites in the stranger, as much as the stranger might, in a perfect world, invite in the mother.

Although communicated via digital media, brelfies exemplify the embodiment of hospitality, connecting subjects and building communities through sharing everyday self-portraiture. Practical and material support for breastfeeding mothers is still needed. So, too, is acceptance that motherwork is profoundly and sometimes spectacularly embodied. To this end, brelfies promote breastfeeding's social value, wherever it may occur.

References

Angiers, N. (1999) *Woman: An intimate geography*, New York: Random House.

Bandura, A. (1982) 'Self-efficacy mechanism in human agency', *American Psychologist*, 37(2): 122–47.

Bartlett, A. (2005) *Breastwork: Rethinking breastfeeding*, Sydney: University of New South Wales Press.

Boon, S. and Pentney, B. (2015) 'Virtual lactivism: breastfeeding selfies and the performance of motherhood', *International Journal of Communication*, 9: 1759–74.

Britton, C. (2009) 'Breastfeeding: a natural phenomenon or a cultural construct?', in C. Squire (ed) *The social context of birth*, Oxford: Radcliff Publishing, pp 305–17.

Bueskens, P. (2015) 'Breastfeeding "in public": a person and political memoir', in L. Raith, J. Jones, M. Porter et al (eds) *Mothers at the margins: Stories of challenge, resistance and love*, Newcastle upon Tyne: Cambridge Scholars Publishing, pp 204–24.

Buzzfeed (2015) 'Facebook Press Release', 4 March, https://www.buzzfeed.com/emaoconnor/brelfies?utm_term=.gtyxOZ5qb#.ji8e7PvMB

Campo, M. (2010) 'The lactating body and conflicting ideals of sexuality, motherhood, and self', in R. Shaw and A. Bartlett (eds) *Giving breastmilk: Body ethics and contemporary breastfeeding practice*, Bradford, ON: Demeter Press, pp 51–63.

Douglas, M. (2002) [1966] *Purity and danger: An analysis of the concepts of pollution and taboo*, London: Routledge.

Doshier, M. (2015) 'The effects of breastfeeding and breastfeeding in public: looking at nursing nooks', [BSci dissertation], California Polytechnic State University.

Dowling, S., Naidoo, J. and Pontin, D. (2012) 'Breastfeeding in public: women's bodies, women's milk', in P. H. Smith, B. L. Hausman and M. Labbok (eds) *Beyond health, beyond choice: Breastfeeding constraints and realities*, New Brunswick, NJ: Rutgers University Press, pp. 249–58.

Freeman, B., Potente, S., Rock, V. and McIver, J. (2015) 'Social media campaigns that make a difference: what can public health learn from the corporate sector and other social change marketers?', *Public Health Research and Practice*, 25(2): e2521517.

Friedman, M. (2013) *Mommyblogs and the changing face of motherhood*, Toronto: University of Toronto Press.

Gibbs Vengrow, B. (nd) 'Alyssa Milano's breastfeeding selfie has nursing moms fired up', https://www.parents.com/baby/all-about-babies/alyssa-milanos-breastfeeding-selfie-has-nursing-moms-fired-up/

Giles, F. (2004) '"Relational and strange": a preliminary foray into a project to queer breastfeeding', *Australian Feminist Studies*, 19(45): 301–14.

Gribble, K. (2005) 'Breastfeeding a medically fragile foster child', *Journal of Human Lactation*, 21(1): 42–6.

Hamilton, P. (2017) 'The "good" attached mother: an analysis of postmaternal and postracial thinking in birth and breastfeeding policy in neoliberal Britain', *Australian Feminist Studies*, 31(90): 410–31.

Hamington, M. (2004) *Embodied care: Jane Addams, Maurice Merleau-Ponty, and feminist ethics*, Chicago, IL: University of Illinois Press.

Hanisch, C. (1970) 'The personal is political', in *Notes from the second year: Women's liberation*, New York: New York Radical Women, p 76.

Hausman, B. (2003) *Mother's milk: Breastfeeding controversies in American culture*, New York: Routledge.

Hausman, B. (2004) 'The feminist politics of breastfeeding', *Australian Feminist Studies*, 19(45): 273–86.

Hausman, B. (2012) 'Feminism and breastfeeding: rhetoric, ideology and the material realities of women's lives', in P. H. Smith, B. L. Hausman and M. Labbok (eds) *Beyond health, beyond choice: Breastfeeding constraints and realities*, New Brunswick, NJ: Rutgers University Press, pp 15–24.

Held, V. (2006) *The ethics of care: Personal, political, and global*, Oxford: Oxford University Press.

Hird, M. (2007) 'The corporeal generosity of maternity', *Body and Society*, (13)1: 1–20.

Hrdy, S. (1999) *Mother nature: Maternal instincts and how they shape the human species*, New York: Ballantine.

Huffington Post (2013) 'Naked breastfeeding yoga mom says that photo was not staged', *Huffington Post*, https://www.huffingtonpost.com/2013/08/20/naked-breastfeeding-yoga-mom_n_3786216.html

Kenny, K. (2016) 'First-person narratives and third-wave feminism: Raising consciousness or the mother of a guilt trip?' [MA dissertation], Macquarie University.

Kirwan-Taylor, H. (2016) 'The rise of the "Brelfie": how breastfeeding selfies became the new way for celebrity mothers to show off', *Daily Mail*, 8 April, www.dailymail.co.uk/femail/article-3529128/The-rise-Brelfie-breast-feeding-new-way-celebrity-mothers-off.html

Knaak, S. (2005) 'The problem with breastfeeding discourse', *Revue Canadienne, de Santé Publique*, 97(5): 412–14.

Komodiki, E., Kontogeorgou, A., Papastavrou, M., Volaki, P., RMidw, Genitsaridi, S. M. and Iacovidou, N. (2014) 'Breastfeeding in public: a global review of different attitudes towards it', *Journal of Pediatrics and Neonatal Care*, 1(6): 00040–43.

Lacan, J. (2001) [1949] 'The mirror stage as formative of the function of the I as revealed in psychoanalytic experience', *Ecrits: A selection*, trans. Alan Sheridan, London: Routledge, pp 502–9.

Lane, R. (2014) 'Healthy discretion? Breastfeeding and the mutual maintenance of motherhood and public space', *Gender, Place and Culture*, 21(2): 195–210.

Lee, R. (2016) 'Feeding the hungry other: breastfeeding, Levinas and the politics of hunger', *Hypatia*, 31(2): 259–74.

Mahon-Daly, P. and Andrews, G. J. (2002) 'Liminality and breastfeeding: women negotiating space and two bodies', *Health and Place*, 8(2): 61–76.

Manne, A. (2005) *Motherhood: How should we care for our children?* Sydney: Allen and Unwin.

Midberry, J. (2017) 'Photos of breastfeeding in uniform: contesting discourses of masculinity, nationalism, and the military', *Feminist Media Studies*, 17(4): 1–17.

Milano, A. (2014) 'Alyssa Milano reacts to her controversial breastfeeding selfie', *ET*, 4 December, www.etonline.com/news/154704_alyssa_milano_reacts_to_her_controversial_breastfeeding_selfie

O'Connor, E. (2015) 'Mums are posting breastfeeding selfies in response to an anti-brelfie critic', *Buzzfeed*, 4 March, https://www.buzzfeed.com/emaoconnor/brelfies?utm_term=.gtyxOZ5qb#.ji8e7PvMB

Penny, L. (2014) *Unspeakable things: Sex, lies and revolution*, New York: Bloomsbury.

Plummer, K. (2003) *Intimate citizenship: Private decisions and public dialogues*, Seattle, WA: University of Washington Press.

Public Health England (2015) 'New mothers are anxious about breastfeeding in public', 2 November, https://www.gov.uk/government/news/new-mothers-are-anxious-about-breastfeeding-in-public

Ruddick, S. (1989) *Maternal thinking: Towards a politics of peace*, London: The Women's Press.

Saito, Y. (2007) *Everyday aesthetics*, Oxford: Oxford University Press.

Shaw, R. (2004) 'The virtues of cross-nursing and the "Yuk Factor"', *Australian Feminist Studies*, 19(45): 287–99.

Shaw, R. and McBride-Henry, S. (2010) 'Giving breastmilk as being-with', in R. Shaw and A. Bartlett (eds) *Giving breastmilk: Body ethics and contemporary breastfeeding practice*, Bradford, ON: Demeter Press, pp 191–204.

Smyth, L. (2009) 'Intimate citizenship and the right to care: the case of breastfeeding,' in E. Olesky (ed) *Intimate citizenships: Gender, sexuality, politics*, New York: Routledge, pp 118–32.

Stephens, J. (2012) *Confronting post-maternal thinking: Feminism, memory and care*, New York: Columbia University Press.

Stephens, J. (2015) 'Reconfiguring care and family in the era of the "out-sourced self"', *Journal of Family Studies*, 21(3): 1–13.

Tech2 (2015) 'Facebook clarifies its rules about what content it bans', *Tech2*, http://tech.firstpost.com/news-analysis/facebook-clarifies-rules-about-what-content-it-bans-and-why-259134.html

Tiidenberg, K. and Cruz, E.G. (2015) 'Selfies, image and the remaking of the body', *Body and Society*, 21(4): 77–102.

Tugwell, S. (2013) 'Imagining the unimaginable: theorising maternal subjectivity through the representation of breastfeeding' [MA dissertation], University of London.

Van Esterik. P. (2015) 'Commensal circles and the common pot', in S. Kerner, C. Chou and M. Warmind (eds) *Commensality: From everyday food to feast*, London: Bloomsbury, pp 31–42.

Vnuk, H. (2015) 'It's a victory for mums over Facebook. We can now do this', Mamamia.com, 17 March, www.mamamia.com.au/breastfeeding-photos-allowed-on-facebook/

Waterlow, L. (2015) 'Rise of the brelfie: breastfeeding selfies are the latest trend for new mums thanks to stars like Miranda Kerr (but is it just "naked exhibitionism"?)', *Daily Mail*, 26 February, www.dailymail.co.uk/femail/article-2968246/Mums-head-head-brelfie-Morning-breastfeeding-selfies-list-parenting-trends-thanks-stars-like-Miranda-Kerr.html

Wakefield, M, Loken, B. and Hornik, R. (2010) 'Use of mass media campaigns to change health behaviour', *Lancet*, 376(9748): 1261–71.

White, A. (2014) 'Facebook removed this mother's picture of her breastfeeding her premature baby because it was "offensive"', *Buzzfeed*, 30 October, https://www.buzzfeed.com/alanwhite/facebook-removed-this-mothers-picture-of-her-breastfeeding-h?utm_term=.dmde2B22X#.prPKj9jj0

Yalom, M. (1997) *A history of the breast*, New York: Knopf.

Yatawara, C. J., Einfeld, S. L. Hickie, I. B., Davenport, T. A. and Guastella, A. J. (2016) 'The effect of oxytocin nasal spray on social interaction deficits observed in young children with autism: a randomized clinical crossover trial', *Molecular Psychiatry*, 21: 1225–31.

ELEVEN

Encountering public art: monumental breasts and the Skywhale

Alison Bartlett

Introduction

This chapter is grounded in the idea that more visual imagery of breastfeeding will contribute to its normalisation, and counter the commercial sexualisation of breasts. I suggest, however, that this strategy is not just about seeing but also about feeling. To demonstrate this I turn to a controversial piece of public art – Patricia Piccinini's Skywhale – which was launched in Australia in 2013 and has been touring internationally. The Skywhale is a hot-air balloon in the shape of a fantastical creature of the imagination, which features five giant breasts on each side. This unexpected flying mammal provokes responses wherever it goes, and arguably provides productive ways of engaging public responses to breastfeeding and maternity. In this chapter I examine responses to Skywhale through broadsheet and social media, and then analyse its affective domain through psychoanalytic concepts and its materiality through the tradition of public art and monuments. The extremes of intimacy and monumentality configured through Skywhale offer an object par excellence for seeing breastfeeding writ large in the public domain, and for feeling the return of the maternal. This, I argue, is fundamental to a shift in perceiving breasts as maternal, and breastfeeding as normative.

Debates around breastfeeding in public often rest on a perceived dichotomy between sexualised breasts being an accepted and ubiquitous aspect of public visual culture, and baby-feeding breasts being an apparently unacceptable – because unusual – public sight and therefore a spectacle. Garland-Thomson reminds us that despite a long cultural history of maternal breasts being 'on view', they have now 'almost entirely receded from view': 'We expect maternal breasts to be sequestered in private spaces whereas erotic breasts are unremarkable staples of public visual culture' (Garland-Thomson, 2009: 143). To gauge the impact of seeing breastfeeding, Hoddinott et al (2010) developed a 'Seeing Breastfeeding' scale to examine the relation between women's reaction to seeing breastfeeding and their likelihood of breastfeeding their babies. From their study of over 400 women in Scotland they found that 'the most important predictor of intending to breastfeed was the woman's attitude to her most recent experience of seeing breastfeeding' (Hoddinott et al, 2010: 134). A more recent study of 254 participants in Canada by Vieth et al measured the impact of women viewing positive breastfeeding posters. They concluded that 'seeing suitable posters can improve the acceptance of seeing a mother breastfeeding in public places' (Vieth et al, 2015: 179).

While Kukla (2006) and Hausman (2007) note that posters can also be condescending and inhibiting, the idea of seeing breastfeeding being modelled is widely understood to be an important indicator of imaging oneself breastfeeding. Drawing on a 2004 report from New South Wales Health, Australia, which found that only 1.3% of 334 articles on breastfeeding contained an image of a breastfeeding baby, Giles concludes that 'there are so few images of women breastfeeding, so few opportunities for people to observe breastfeeding women, to learn about breastfeeding through incidental exposure, and to consider it commonplace' (Giles, 2012: 1). Boyer also notes that public space still needs to be recoded as a place where baby-feeding breasts are normal, and she notes the way that contemporary lactivism and breastfeeding picnics 'seek to change norms around how urban space is understood … rescripting an activity coded as intimate and belonging in the space of the home as being equally appropriate in public space' (Boyer, 2011: 434). These contestations of space can be understood as troubling, deeply ingrained understandings of women's 'place' in public and private spheres. Linked to demographic shifts, when women are having fewer children later in life it means that we, as both babies and adults, are unaccustomed to seeing maternal breasts. These underlying factors exert a profoundly enduring force on social practices of breastfeeding.

Drawing on this field of research, this chapter looks at the ways that public art might participate in recoding space, in drawing attention to maternal breasts through art and therefore as an acceptable occupier of space, thus contributing to seeing breasts in public that are not (just) sexualised. The Skywhale (2013) is a useful piece to investigate because it is so big, so controversial, and unmistakably all about maternal breasts. I'm particularly interested in the idea of affect – how people react, what they feel and how this might be understood psychosocially – and in materiality – how objects take up and refigure space, how materials and size work, and how we interact with those factors. The materiality I'm discussing is not necessarily about 'real' breasts, but rather their symbolic manifestation and the responses they provoke through public art. And yet it is also about 'real' breasts, because public responses are inextricably connected to the meanings we attach to breastfeeding as a social practice and a personal experience. My argument is that encountering artworks like the Skywhale renders maternal breasts visible in public places. Removed from conventional breastfeeding contexts, such encounters with public art are inextricably tied to our feelings about breastfeeding and the maternal.

Skywhale

The Skywhale is a work by Australian artist Patricia Piccinini, commissioned for an occasion: the Centenary of Canberra. Canberra is Australia's capital city and the location of Federal Parliament; it is a city specifically designed for that purpose by architect Walter Burley Griffin. The centenary marks 100 years since it was named by Lady Denham, whose husband was the Governor General; this post-holder is the Queen's representative in Australia. It might seem strange to have a capital city that is only 100 years old, so in this respect the strange, ancient, fantastical creature that is the Skywhale is oddly apt for the occasion. Since the centenary event in March 2013, Skywhale has turned up at music and art festivals in at least three other Australian cities and two regional towns, and has been hired for similar events and festivals in Japan, Ireland and Brazil.

While a work of imagination, Skywhale references the fanciful evolution of the whale into a sky-dwelling rather than sea-dwelling mammal. In the form of a hot-air balloon, the creature has a broad, dark back; a tail resembling that of a platypus; and a benign, ancient-looking face that resembles a turtle. Five drooping pinkish breasts hang from each side, and an underbelly falls to the balloon's basket. The scale of this creature is massive, so that the basket in which people can ride is insignificant in many images of the balloon. To provide an idea of its scale, one of the formal descriptions includes the following information about its material composition:

> Skywhale is a sculpture, a special shaped hot air balloon conceived by Patricia Piccinini and built by Cameron Balloons in the United Kingdom. The colours, patterns and textures have been carefully printed onto 3,535 metres of fabric. She was cut and sewn together by a team

of six people using approximately 3.3 million stitches! The Skywhale is an Australian Registered aircraft. She is controlled by a pilot and is operated under the Australian Standards pertaining to aviation. When inflated she stands 24 metres high and is 36 metres in length.

Piccinini talks about the Skywhale as a wondrous creature, a reminder of the miracles of nature, the chances of evolutionary design, and our capacity to relate to other creatures, our relation to nature, and to strangeness (Pearce, 2013).

Media reactions

As a piece of public art commissioned for an occasion, Skywhale has predictably been controversial. In the words of the Centenary artistic director Robyn Archer:

> Skywhale had to run the predictable gauntlet of mass media mischief, 'public funding' outrage, violent opinion from many who had never seen the work, and 'what's it got to do with Canberra?' until this marvelous work established itself as a huge favourite of people all over Australia and the world, and almost as a symbol of Canberra's bold adventurous aspect. (Archer, 2013: 6)

This is perhaps an optimistic view from a director. Cartoonists certainly derived much pleasure in relating it to 'teat-sucking rent-seekers, hot-air-filled media personalities and political Captain Ahabs', as well-known Canberra Times cartoonist David Pope so eloquently puts it (Pope, 2013). Similarly, media editors were able to concoct headlines like:

> 'Skywhale: Success story or a big boob?' (Jean and Page, 2013)

> 'Libs fuming over "Hindenboob disaster"' (Jean, 2013)

> 'Crippled nipples a sag state of affairs' (Hannaford and Thomson, 2014)

> 'Skywhale to titillate Newcastle' (McMahon, 2014)

Controversy was courted most publicly when one city councillor in Tasmania called it 'suggestive and offensive to women', because 'there were 16 great breasts hanging down … and it was on display for anybody to see' (ABC News, 2013). As indicated by the hyperbole of increasing the number of breasts to 16 in this report, it was Skywhale's mammaries that caused most controversy and snickering. On the (now defunct) Skywhale website, however, Robyn Archer insisted that people 'were won over by the sheer size, the skill of workmanship, and the creature's benign, maternal, presence'.

Indications of people having been won over emerged in social media as the hashtag #skywhale gained momentum. People are inspired to create their own replicas, implying some sort of adoption, or mirroring, or at least acceptance into the imaginary of their world. There are playful images posted on Twitter, Instagram and Facebook of crocheted skywhale headwear, and another bonnet made of balloons, a papier mâché model, skywhale cakes and cupcakes, plasticine models, glasswork replicas, a skywhale made of Lego, and people posing beside skywhale street art. People notice skywhale in their bocconcini, and in mammatus clouds, which are hashtagged to Skywhale, and there's an ode to Skywhale uploaded to the music site Bandcamp. Piccinini mentions in an interview at the Museum of Old and New Art (MONA), Tasmania, that Skywhale has not only become a meme, but a 'thing', as when someone tweeted during the Eurovision contest, 'This is boring. It needs more skywhale' (Pearce, 2013). The advantage of scanning social media is that it provides a countermedia to traditional and often conservative print media. While the division of responses as I've reported them here are not so neatly divided into appalling and appealing, there is certainly a playfulness and curiosity about Skywhale evident on social media that is noticeably absent in the more formal news media. To explore the potency of this particular piece of public art, I investigate Skywhale on two scales: through considering its monumental size and its intimate psychic relations.

Analysing affect

The reactions to Skywhale seem to be polarised into no and yes, fear and wonder, strangeness and familiarity, rejection and embrace, and perhaps *fort-da* (gone-there). *Fort-da* is the name Freud gave to the game of disappearance and retrieval, when he observed his grandson – the little Ernst – hiding his toys and then finding them again, and then in his cot throwing away a wooden cotton reel on a string and then retrieving it. Freud proposed that this was the infant's way of relinquishing the mother. The game is understood to be an exercise of imagined control. As Freud writes in 'Beyond the pleasure principle':

> It was related to the child's great cultural achievement – the instinctual renunciation (that is, the renunciation of instinctual satisfaction) which he had made in allowing his mother to go away without protesting. (Freud, 1961 [1920]: 14–15)

Later developments in psychoanalysis by object-relations theorists proposed that the renunciation of the mother is too simple an explanation to account for the acquisition of subjectivity, and criticised the model for being based solely on a boy-child. Freud also came to realise that the mother–child relation might be different for girls. As an antidote to this, Klein proposed that these complex emotional relations were focused around objects and their internationalisation as phantasy. Klein proposes the breast as the first love object, but in no benign or simple relation. Rather, she contends a complex and predominantly hostile relation as the breast becomes split into the good and bad breast, depending on whether it is available or not in sync with the child's wishes. The process of reconciling the absence of the breast becomes the psychic terrain on which the child works through anxieties and frustrations as well as needs and desires. It might seem fanciful to use these slithers of psychoanalytic theory to think about the effects of a piece of public art like Skywhale. And yet, how can those encounters be anything but responses to the reappearance of the maternal breast after all this time? And so many? And so big? Not only to return, but in excess, in plentitude.

The expressions on social media, which tend towards the almost inarticulate 'wow' to inadequate reaches of excess, are perhaps symptomatic of these complex emotional relations, which find themselves irrupting in almost preverbal language. I heard an announcer on ABC Radio National (the Australian equivalent to BBC Radio 4) introduce Piccinini on air and begin stumbling over his script and adlibbing in an effort to render something of the Skywhale's reputation. This is Michael Cathcart, in his sonorous radio voice:

> 'Piccinini creates very unsettling life-size hybrid sculptures that are a comment on our relationship with nature. Her latest is the Skywhale. I suppose it's a sculpture, it's really a balloon. It's this hot-air balloon, that's in the shape of an otherworldly creature. It looks more like a giant big turtle

to me than a whale, but it has these [pause] pendulous udders, these [pause] great breasts that hang down along the sides and when you look up in the sky there are these [pause] bosoms looming over you as this thing makes its way through the atmosphere. It's very stunning indeed.' (Cathcart, 2015)

When he departs from the script he slows down and emphasises words, leaves gaps, repeats himself, says the same thing using different words, as if language becomes inadequate; as if the gaps and gestures, the sounds and rhythms are more expressive in describing Skywhale. As if Skywhale invokes the semiotic.

In psychoanalytic theories of the child's development, the entry into language is the most significant transition in becoming a speaking subject, and is considered to be a shift from the maternal world to the father's. In Lacan's reworking of Freud's theories, he terms the realm of language, culture and ideas, the symbolic. The Symbolic governs us as speaking subjects through language, logic, law and order, which Lacan terms the Law of the Father. Kristeva's reworking of Lacan's ideas reinstates the value of the maternal through the primary relation to the mother during the pre-symbolic phase, the pre-Oedipal, or what Kristeva termed the Semiotic. The Semiotic is characterised by pulsations, rhythm, intonation, gesture – it is the prelinguistic realm. For the speaking subject to emerge, they must inevitably leave behind the Semiotic, but Kristeva maintains that it remains, threatening to erupt through the Symbolic, and is identifiable in moments of poetry, or else in psychosis. These are disruptive forces, she insists, because they threaten the illusion of symbolic language as fixed and stable – as understandable. Indeed, they threaten the illusion of ourselves as understandable (Kristeva, 1984; Boulous Walker, 1998; Beuskins, 2014). There is something profoundly affecting happening when those primal prelinguistic patterns become forces of speech.

Monumentalism

Those expressions of excess are commensurate with the physical scale of Skywhale, which can be thought about through the tradition of the monument. Stewart suggests that the size of objects has a history in the public imagination: 'We find the miniature at the origin of private, individual history, but we find the gigantic at the origin of public and natural history' (Stewart, 1993: 71). The public monument is usually located in cities, and in these sites of dense systems of representation, they stand up and out over their landscape. We see this in the official video clips of Skywhale, like the one titled 'In her natural habitat' (Balharrie, 2013), where Skywhale moves over and through the landscape. It is significant that her natural habitat is Canberra and its surrounds. This is the place and event of the commission, but Canberra is also the site of Australia's archives and historical legacies, with 11 national institutions residing there, including the National Museum of Australia, National Library of Australia, National Gallery of Australia, National Archives of Australia, National Portrait Gallery and the Australian War Memorial, as well as Federal Parliament. Indeed, this city can be understood as not only housing, but also generative of, democracy, arts, archives, objects. In this sense, the work of Skywhale is also monumental, and yet in her natural habitat it is often the landscape that dwarfs her. Monuments are figured through other aspects of their materiality: they are usually impressively solid, immovable, heavy, made of weighty and often classical earthly materials like marble, steel or wood. Skywhale is much more aligned with the element of air: its fabric is soft and billowy, it is filled with air, sometimes fired by a flare of gas, it moves, it is prone to deflating and transient. It is ethereal and ephemeral.

Skywhale differs from public art in being untethered, moving across locations. Hein points out a shift in public art during the late twentieth century when it came down from its pedestal into a more engaged, grassroots participatory sphere, due to its locations:

> Public art, unlike the more sequestered private art, appears in pedestrian places, like playgrounds and shopping malls, along highways and the ordinary junctures of life. Even when its purpose is to celebrate heroism and transcendence, it aims to speak to common people and is meant to bring them together. (Hein, 2006: xxii)

A function of monuments and public art has traditionally been to lend authority and longevity to heroic figures and historical events, to display their significance through size and verticality. Piccinini talks about ruling out the expectation that she might make a giant head of Canberra's designer Burley-Griffin (Pearce, 2013). Monuments traditionally honour death: they are temples to warriors, soldiers, mythical and real battles, slain dragons, kings, emperors, and empires. Their size partly functions to amplify their status in history, and this is enhanced by dwarfing the viewer in what Stewart calls the removal of the transcendental position. She explains that, in contrast to the vast scale of history and heroism, we are in comparison slight, and compelled 'to acknowledge the fallen, the victorious, the heroic, and be taken up in the history of place' (Stewart, 1993: 90). In stark contrast, the scale of Skywhale doesn't function to heroise or historicise, but rather asks of us something more personal, even inflating the personal and our commonality in being born and mothered. Piccinini says, 'I could have made something quite scary, but I went to great lengths to make her very benign. She's got a very beatific smile, she's very Buddha-like, she's calm and gentle' (Arts Today, 2013). Rather than removing a transcendental position of sovereignty, perhaps Skywhale reinstalls the viewer to the position of infant through a maternal gaze.

Scariness is something often evoked by giants in fairytale and myth, and Stewart notes that giants are often male, devouring and cannibalistic (1993: 88). When women are occasionally giants, it is their bodies that become the focus of monstrosity, especially their breasts. She reminds us of Swift's second book of Gulliver's Travels, when Gulliver is in Brobdingnag, the land of giants, where the women have terrifying, gigantic, diseased breasts that threaten to engulf and swallow Gulliver (Stewart, 1993). You might also recall Philip Roth's book The breast (1972), where an aging male literature professor inexplicably and terrifyingly turns into a giant breast. These stifling and devouring breast stories contrast the Skywhale, whose scale seems to work benevolently. Piccinini links scale with benevolence when she says, 'I think it's quite an emotional work. To have this huge gargantuan and benign figure come down on you is quite affecting' (Arts Today, 2013).

Connections

The monumental size of Skywhale and the onslaught of responses, whether for or against, are testament to the impact of Skywhale as a piece of public art. Piccinini insists that she wants people to be moved by the installation, that as a commission for a public sculpture she had 'an obligation to make an object that people could really connect with' (Pearce, 2013). This is consistent with all her work, which is often described as probing what it means to be human in a contemporary biotech posthuman world (Toffoletti, 2003), and she typically refers to feelings and emotions as a way of inviting viewers to think about her ideas.

While she doesn't target maternity per se, Piccinini's installations are interested in our place in the world and relations between creatures, which involves relations of caring, responsibility, love and parenting. The Young Family (2002), for example, humanises a suckling sow and her babies while also making strange that humanness. The borders between human and animal unhinge, and the gallery didactics tell us is was made in response to the breeding of genetically modified pigs to provide replacement organs and cells for humans, suggesting a more sinister ethical relation. Big Mother (2005) is an ape-like creature suckling a human-like baby with an uncannily maternal expression. It is 1.75 metres high, made from silicone, fibreglass, leather and human hair: its materiality is at once human, animal and technological, inserted in the midst of these worlds. Piccinini recounts two origin stories for Big Mother: the first in South Africa, where she met someone whose baby sister had been taken by a grieving baboon to replace the animal's baby; the second when Piccinini was having trouble breastfeeding, and her sister offered up her own six-month-old baby to teach her how to do it (Ireland, 2012). The cross-species and cross-family breastfeeding practices are congealed in an artwork that invites emotional responses and their consequences for how we treat each other and other beings in the world. Piccinini's interest in care relations, maternity and breastfeeding, and in posthuman biotechnology, speciesism and evolutionary wonders, are all evident in Skywhale, and ask us to consider our maternal relations and mammalian breasted-ness.

Artist and psychoanalyst Bracha L. Ettinger proposes that art has a very special relation to the maternal, through what she names the matrixial. Not content with the theories of subject formation that relegate the mother to a lost object, to a thing that we need to separate from or cleft against, Ettinger proposes another forgotten, more archaic, relation that is established prior to birth and which lays down a psychic sphere of relationality where we encounter each other in the same body. In utero, she claims, is a space and a time of 'transgressive encounter between I and non-I grounded in the maternal womb/intra-uterine complex and a notion of affective economy that avoids phallocentrism' (Ettinger, 2006: 218). The womb/matrix is not necessarily an organ or an origin but 'the human potentiality for difference-in-co-emergence' (2006: 219). It is a trans-subjective space that lays the groundwork for encounters with Others throughout life. Ettinger calls this the matrixial borderspace, where 'subjectivity here is an encounter between I and un-cognized yet intimate non-I neither rejected nor assimilated' (p 218). She asks us to conceive this encounter as 'traces of links, trans-individual transmissions and transformational reattunements, rather than of relations to and communication with objects and subjects' (p 220). And the matrixial, she claims, 'draws a special connection between analytical practice as an ethical working-through and artistic practice as an aesthetical working-through'. Ethical and aesthetical compassion are key to the continuing passage of the matrixial in a process she calls metramorphosis, which operates not instead of but alongside phallic psychoanalytic models 'on a different unconscious track' (p 220).

I find Ettinger's theories suggestive and potent for an argument that encountering public art can be a transformative space for the normalisation of breastfeeding. For Ettinger, art is a form of therapy: it reminds us of the links between aesthetics and ethics, and our relations to each other in the world, that were established in utero, and that, despite all our trying through misogyny or matricide, or even just disavowing the mother or the maternal, it still exists as the primary state of our being. Ettinger invents a language to talk about this because there is no language, and Piccinini's artwork manifests this in provocative and powerful ways that are not necessarily conscious nor able to be easily expressed.

Both Ettinger and Piccinini suggest that art should move us, and when this happens we are touched by reminders about our place in the world, our relationality to others. The primal relation between mother and baby is of interest to both artists. I'm reminded of the response of a Tasmanian woman who got to ride in the basket of Skywhale and was interviewed on local ABC radio in Launceston. She was marvelling not only at the "bird's eye view", but in being able "to see up inside Skywhale" as she moved through the sky. She tells the reporter in a soft, slow, wondrous voice:

> 'I have been up in Skywhale. What a wonderful surprise. Very unexpected. Very gentle. Beautiful to just look up at the whole structure from underneath there … I never would have thought a week or two ago that I could say I've been in Skywhale. Very exciting.' (Walker, 2013)

This arresting image of being in Skywhale is reminiscent of being inside the womb/matrix, where the balloon basket becomes a threshold space of matrixial borderlinks. The art historian Griselda Pollock takes up Ettinger's insistence on aesthetic affect when she says:

> Here we might find ways to think not only subjectivity in this abstracted theoretical form, but aesthetic encounters of viewers and art works, and also ethical and political relations between strange, foreign, irreducible elements of otherness in our encounters with human and even non-human events in the world. (Pollock, 2004: 7)

Pollock's thinking is joined to Ettinger's politics about how we relate to enemies, to what is foreign, to refugees and the dispossessed, to the strangeness of future technologies as well as the inexplicability of the past: for example, imagining if the whale had become a sky-dwelling mammal rather than an air-breathing sea-dweller. In this sense, maternal relations are considered to lay down the model for all future relations in the world. Normalising breastfeeding becomes not only the most effective form of nutrition for babies, but a reminder of our inextricable link to all others on the planet through the originary maternal relation.

Conclusion

I've argued here that Skywhale is an affective piece of public art that touches some primal relation to the archaic maternal, primarily due to its spectacular mammalian breasts. In trying to articulate this, I've drawn on a discourse of psychoanalysis, which is an unwieldy and in many ways unsatisfactory language, which is why Ettinger creates so many new terms. But it is no more unwieldy than medicine and public health, which presently have authoritative dominion over explanations of breastfeeding and its meanings. Encounters with artworks like Skywhale, I suggest, are affective and therefore effective in reviving feelings about breastfeeding that prompt webs of connections, separation-in-jointness, border-linking encounters (Ettinger, 2006). They provide another form of encounter with maternal breasts and may prompt another form of language to articulate that primary relation, whether through preverbal expression or playful and creative responses in crochet, music or baking. As Ahmed suggests, objects that move us, that create a movement of emotion, become affective; and emotions are what move us into life, while also holding us in place, connecting us to things, to places, to others, to ourselves (Ahmed, 2004: 11). This is monumental indeed.

References
ABC News (2013) 'Skywhale degrading and offensive, says Tasmanian alderman', *ABC News*, www.abc.net.au/news/2013-06-25/tasmanian-alderman-labels-skywhale-degrading/4777904

Ahmed, S. (2004) *The cultural politics of emotion*, Edinburgh: Edinburgh University Press.

Archer, R. (2013) 'Centenary chronicle chapter 1', *Australian Journal of Music Education*, 2: 3–16.

Arts Today (2013) 'Skywhale prompts an emotional reaction to difficult things: Patricia Piccinini', ABC Radio National, www.abc.net.au/arts/stories/s3762859.htm

Balharrie, S. (dir.) (2013) 'In her natural habitat', Skywhale official promotional video, https://www.youtube.com/watch?v=kWKeTOYudzo

Beuskins, P. (2014) 'Introduction', in P. Beuskins (ed) *Mothering and psychoanalysis: Clinical, sociological and feminist perspectives*, Toronto: Demeter Press, pp 1–72.

Boulous Walker, M. (1998) *Philosophy and the maternal body: Reading silence*, London: Routledge.

Boyer, K. (2011) '"The way to break the taboo is to do the taboo thing": breastfeeding in public and citizen-activism in the UK', *Health and Place*, 17: 430–37.

Cathcart, M. (2015) 'Top Shelf: Patricia Piccinini', *ABC Radio National*, www.abc.net.au/radionational/programs/booksandartsdaily/top-shelf3a-patricia-piccinini/6048468

Ettinger, B. L. (2006) 'Matrixial trans-subjectivity', *Theory, Culture and Society*, 23(2–3):218–22.

Freud, S. (1961) [1920] *Beyond the pleasure principle*, London: Hogarth Press and the Institute of Psycho-Analysis.

Garland-Thomson, R. (2009) *Staring: How we look*, New York: Oxford University Press.

Giles, F. (2012) 'Time #3: why does it hurt to look at a woman breastfeeding?', *The Conversation*, https://theconversation.com/time-3-why-does-it-hurt-to-look-at-a-woman-breastfeeding-7066

Hannaford, S. and Thomson, P. (2014) 'Crippled nipples a sag state of affairs', The Canberra Times, 9 March, available through Factiva.

Hausman, B. L. (2007) 'Things (not) to do with breasts in public: maternal embodiment and the biocultural politics of infant feeding', *New Literary History*, 38(3): 479–504.

Hein, H. S. (2006) *Public art: Thinking museums differently*, Oxford: AltaMira Press.

Hoddinott, P., Kroll, T., Raja, A. and Lee, A. J. (2009) 'Seeing other women breastfeed: how vicarious experience relates to breastfeeding intention and behaviour', *Maternal and Child Nutrition*, 6: 134–46.

Ireland, P. (2012) 'A talk with artist Patricia Piccinini, whose disquieting yet appealing works explore the bond between man and animal', *Nashville Scene*, www.nashvillescene.com/arts-culture/article/13042697/a-talk-with-artist-patricia-piccinini-whose-disquieting-yet-appealing-works-explore-the-bond-between-man-and-animal

Jean, P. (2013) 'Libs fuming over "Hindenboob disaster"', *The Canberra Times*, www.canberratimes.com.au/act-news/libs-fuming-over-hindenboob-disaster-20130514-2jk1s.html

Jean, P. and Page, F. (2013) 'Skywhale: success story or a big boob?', *The Canberra Times*, www.canberratimes.com.au/act-news/skywhale-success-story-or-a-big-boob-20130514-2jkyn.html

Kristeva, J. (1984) *Revolution in poetic language*, New York: Columbia University Press.

Kukla, R. (2006) 'Ethics and ideology in breastfeeding advocacy campaigns', *Hypatia*, 21(1): 157–80.

McMahon, J. (2014) 'Skywhale to titillate Newcastle', 1233 ABC Newcastle, www.abc.net.au/local/photos/2014/10/27/4115496.htm

Pearce E. (2013) 'Interview with the Skywhale artist Patricia Piccinini', *MONA Blog*, http://monablog.net/2013/06/22/interview-with-skywhale-artist-patricia-piccinini/

Pollock, G. (2004) 'Thinking the feminine: aesthetic practice as introduction to Bracha Ettinger and the concepts of matrix and metramorphosis', *Theory, Culture and Society*, 21(1): 5–65.

Pope, D. (2013) 'David Pope reflects on Canberra in 2013', *Sydney Morning Herald*, www.smh.com.au/comment/david-pope-reflects-on-canberra-in-2013-20131219-2zozn.html

Roth, P. (1972) The breast, New York: Houghton Mifflin Harcourt.

Stewart, S. (1993) [1984] *On longing: Narratives of the miniature, the gigantic, the souvenir, the collection*, Durham, NC: Duke University Press.

Toffoletti, K. (2003) 'Imagining the posthuman: Patricia Piccinini and the art of simulation', *Outskirts*, 11, www.outskirts.arts.uwa.edu.au/volumes/volume-11/toffoletti

Vieth, A., Woodrow, J., Murphy-Goodridge, J., O'Neil, C. and Roebothan, B. (2015) 'The ability of posters to enhance the comfort level with breastfeeding in a public venue in rural Newfoundland and Labrador', *Journal of Human Lactation*, 32(1): 174–81.

Walker, T. (2013) 'Skywhale skirts controversy in Launceston', *ABC Northern Tasmania*, www.abc.net.au/local/videos/2013/06/25/3789092.htm

TWELVE

Embodiment as a gauge of individual, public and planetary health

Maia Boswell-Penc

Introduction

In 2016 the *Lancet* published a series of papers showcasing the importance of situating breastfeeding within its social and cultural contexts (Rollins et al, 2016; Victora et al, 2016). I begin this chapter by considering the specific context of the workplace, as it presents significant barriers to women seeking to continue breastfeeding as they return to work (Boswell-Penc and Boyer, 2007). I move from there to consider lactating working mothers alongside lactating (working) cows, the source of most infant formula that non-nursing mothers use. Considering both lactating mothers and lactating cows, I find that increasing degrees of embodiment correspond with increasing degrees of individual, public and planetary health.

I assume here the broadest social and cultural view, as we reside at a precipice in terms of public health (Fuhrman, 2003; Weber, 2009) as well as climate change and global depletion (IPCC, 2014). Breast milk for young ones and non-dairy milk for others emerges as critical to securing optimal health for all; additionally, as research has surfaced pointing to ways in which we make healthier decisions when we focus on others, compassion becomes an entry into moving into practices that support global health (Poulin, 2013). As research into 'kangaroo care' – skin-to-skin engagement with infants – suggests, full embodiment increases compassion, just as breastfeeding increases oxytocin (Ludington-Hoe and Swinth, 1996). Compassion in its broadest sense may become part of the toolbox that can help breastfeeding professionals make a case for exclusive and extended breastfeeding.

Barriers, embodiment and disembodiment

A few years ago, Kate Boyer and I conducted research into barriers that prevent mothers from continuing to breastfeed after their return to work (Boswell-Penc and Boyer, 2007). In addition to the legal and logistical barriers, a surprising barrier that we encountered was women's perceptions of themselves using breast pumps. Many said that the thought of using the devices made them 'feel like a cow' (Boswell-Penc and Boyer, 2007). They were anxious that the activity might leave them feeling disembodied, not like themselves, but rather like a cow in the dairy industry. Cows' lives in these contexts, after all, are hyper-focused around milk production, often with grave consequences (Webster, 1986; Foer, 2009). Whatever the source of anxiety, these women opted for formula use upon returning to work after maternity leave (Boswell-Penc and Boyer, 2007).

The fear that being hooked to a pump can render one somehow cut off from one's body and baby brings us to more pronounced scenes of disembodiment. More specifically, lactating mothers who are unable or unwilling to breastfeed their children upon resuming work bring us to a looming truth (Boswell-Penc and Boyer, 2007). The use of infant formula represents disembodiment as we leave the arena of even partial embodiment (as with expressing milk for later use) and enter the domain of simulation. Synthetic, corporate, controlled mechanisms of nutrition rule the day but the link between lactating women and lactating cows brings us to other juxtapositions.

We can locate three scenes. First, we encounter the scene of full embodiment, where mothers breastfeed their infants. Second, we witness the scene of partial embodiment of breast pumps, where a third party bottle-feeds breast milk. Finally, we get to the scene lacking embodiment, where children receive infant formula from a bottle. Here mothers are no longer tied to their children in the same way and mothers' bodies are no longer life-sustaining in the same way.

Freely provided and freely distributed, mother's milk is best suited for human infants (Scariati et al, 1997; Goldman, 2000). We must keep in mind that formula use requires water, packaging, advertising and transportation, thus draining precious resources in the production and distribution stages. In addition, bottle feeding requires plastic, rubber, silicone and glass for bottles and teats, and water, detergent and chemicals for cleaning 'delivery devices'. Bottle feeding, in some ways, becomes the enabler of disembodiment.

In comparison, cows suckling their young represent full embodiment. Vast expanses of concrete-and-dirt spaces which make up the industrial farming system, also called 'factory farms' or 'concentrated animal feeding operations' (CAFOs), where hundreds of thousands of cows remain hooked up to milking machines, many never allowed pasture and enduring repeated pain and infections, constitute often horrific scenes of disembodiment (Scully, 2002; Foer, 2009). This system also supplies most of the infant formula industry, where cows become not so much living, breathing creatures as machines themselves (Grossman, 2014; Mayo Clinic, 2016). Anyone who has seen photos of rows and rows of cows hooked up to milking machines, with concrete and steel having crowded out grass, hay and sunshine, understands this characterisation of CAFOs as 'factory farms'.

So why do I compare these scenes of embodiment, partial embodiment, disembodiment, suckling, pumping and approximated milk? I contend that important truths reveal themselves by considering mothers breastfeeding, pumping and using formula alongside cows suckling and producing milk in the vast, multibillion-dollar dairy industry.

Full embodiment as key to best practices

Comparing these scenes highlights how 'personal habits' and practices interact in particular ways with policies and legislation that take place on a larger, societal level. Similarly, juxtaposing scenes of human feeding and nutrition alongside our bovine counterparts brings us to an important understanding. Both point us towards positive habits and best practices for new mothers, breastfeeding counsellors, peer supporters, public health managers, doulas and midwives. They also point us towards positive habits and best practices for 'factory farming' industries. Indeed, such considerations help us think clearly about our own habits, practices and policies. This is particularly important when we consider not only the public health and environmental effects of using breast milk, infant formula, cows' milk and 'alternative milks,' but also the psychosocial effects of various choices (Steingraber, 2001; Tuttle, 2005; Boswell-Penc, 2006; Foer, 2009). This is about imagining the ideal, because utopian dreaming has its place, particularly at times of crisis.

If the practice of mothers exclusively breastfeeding their children long term evokes notions of full embodiment, so too does the notion of cows suckling their calves set free from the machine and no longer forced to be a cog in the vast industrialised farming system. In a fully embodied world, mothers breastfeed and cows suckle. The upshot? The formula and dairy industries either disappear, or change radically. And the diets of infants and children become healthier. This is significant for the US, UK and other industrialised countries in the global North, where rates of diet-related chronic health conditions such as type 2 diabetes continue to rise (American Diabetic Association, 2003; Fuhrman, 2003; Campbell and Campbell, 2005). This also has significance for much of the rest of the world, because the trends in many countries tend to follow in the footsteps of those carried out in the 'global North' (Ornish, 2003; Harper, 2010).

In this 'utopian' scene of full embodiment, infant formula – the proxy for mother's milk – falls out of the picture. Here human milk banks fill the gaps for children who cannot have their own mothers' milk. In this space of health and full embodiment, alternatives for older children and adults are supplied in the form of 'alternative milks'. While some 'alternatives' come with some environmental and potential health burdens that need to be considered, many have argued for the comparative benefits, particularly of coconut, rice and hemp milk (Gartner, 2005; Oppenlander, 2012). Imagine the benefits for mothers and children as infant formula and dairy are withdrawn from the scene (Fuhrman, 2003; Campbell and Campbell, 2005).

Imagine the health benefits for Earth as human breast milk finally comes to replace the heavy environmental costs associated with the production and distribution of infant formula, including the resource depletion and climate-changing impacts linked to the dairy industry (Foer, 2009; Goodland and Anhang, 2009; Hertwich et al, 2010; Eshel et al, 2014). The fertility-limiting effects of mothers breastfeeding exclusively and long term (Dobson and Murtaugh, 2001) throws the discrepancy into an even more powerful light, particularly as we continue to bump up against the limits of Earth's carrying capacity. Breast milk is 'best' from multiple vantage points (Steingraber, 2001; Boswell-Penc, 2006).

The juxtaposition of breast milk and formula and non-dairy milks (allowing for full embodiment for the cow and her calf) and dairy (associated with disembodiment from the cow's perspective) brings to the forefront ways in which degrees of embodiment and compassion become gauges leading to greater health and wellbeing. Movement away from formula and dairy benefits infants and mothers, as well as cows and their offspring. But when we add the consumption of cow's bodies to the equation, we enter the scene of literal disembodiment. Doing so demonstrates how full embodiment continues to serve as a gauge of human and planetary health. This becomes clearer as research continues to emerge demonstrating the many benefits of a plant-based diet, particularly as rates of obesity, heart disease, diabetes, cancers and other health issues have increased (Yale University, 2001; Fuhrman, 2003; Campbell and Campbell, 2005; Gartner, 2005; Oppenlander, 2012;).

Adding to this trend, bovine growth hormones and antibiotics used in animal feed in the US dairy industry have been associated with human endocrine problems and antibiotic-resistant strains of influenza and other diseases (Wuethrich, 2003; Gartner, 2005). Of note is the fact that in the US 80% of the antibiotics used each year are fed to animals on factory farms to prevent infection and disease, which would spread quickly due to the conditions in which animals are housed (Foer, 2009). The literature and research illustrates the link between the dairy and meat industries in the industrialised factory farming system (Scully, 2002; Tuttle, 2005; Foer, 2009; Oppenlander, 2012), the health benefits of refraining from meat and dairy (Host, 2002; Fuhrman, 2003; Campbell and Campbell, 2005; Gartner, 2005; Oppenlander, 2012), and the psychosocial benefits of full embodiment (Rowe, 1999; Scully, 2002; Tuttle, 2005; Foer, 2009; Harper, 2010).

At the extreme edge of the meat industry's disembodiment practice is the cannibalising of cows where the unwanted carcass bits left over from the beef industry are put back into cows' feed (Scully, 2002; Foer, 2009). This practice may be characterised as taboo (given the forced cannibalism) and as 'disembodiment' in a literal sense, as it seems to stem from the head being cut off from the heart; here I refer not just to the cow's head being cut off from its heart – to the horror of dismemberment, which PETA (People for the Ethical Treatment of Animals) has so well documented (Foer, 2009; Harper, 2010) – but also to the figurative 'head' being cut off from its 'heart'. The phenomenon of 'mad cow disease' (bovine spongiform encephalopathy, or BSE) should make us pause over the madness not of cows but of us humans who would even think of such practices, let alone institute them on such a global scale that millions of innocent cows had to be put to death for fear of the spread of 'mad cow disease' (Scully, 2002).

Environmental issues complicate narratives

I want to consider now the environmental costs that arise from varying scenes of embodiment and disembodiment. If we travel back through time to imagine ourselves on a Sunday morning, 29 March 1970, we might see ourselves sipping a cup of tea and reading the *New York Times*. This is eight years after Rachel Carson published her seminal book *Silent spring*, which alerted people to the consequences of using pesticides and other toxic chemicals in farming, lawn care, household cleaning and personal care (Carson, 1962). Noting the slow pace of the damage, the Environmental Defense Fund (EDF) releases a newspaper advertisement that morning that became the group's first membership campaign (EDF, 2002). Internal EDF documents demonstrate the group's excitement. The campaign seemed to get at a poignant story that EDF felt would bring people to notice the dire effects of our unscrupulous use of toxins (EDF, 2002).

The campaign features a photo of a mother with a child near her breast, and the tag line, 'Is Mother's Milk Fit for Human Consumption?' (EDF, 2002). The logic behind the campaign went like this: 'If this most pristine of substances is tainted with toxins, isn't that the perfect wake-up call?' (Boswell-Penc, 2006). Unfortunately, the message came at an inopportune time, when breastfeeding rates were at a low. The infant formula industry was ratcheting up its campaign and sending countless mothers home from hospitals with free samples. Its literature represented their product as being at least as good as, if not better than, mother's milk (Boswell-Penc, 2006). At the same time, the formula industry had begun its attempt to colonise the global South and much of the 'developing world', with its products administered by salespeople dressed in white medical garb (Boswell-Penc, 2006).

A more problematic issue was that, from the perspective of many breastfeeding advocates, EDF's message seemed too complicated and too dangerous, and was deemed not worth the risk of potentially turning mothers away from breastfeeding (Boswell-Penc, 2006). Surely, it could not be a good thing for mothers sitting at the top of the food chain to discover that their breast milk might possibly carry a toxic load, right? The reality that breast milk is *still* best, except in the rarest cases of supercharged contamination, somehow seemed too unwieldy an argument (Boswell-Penc, 2006).

So the campaign was silenced. Since that day in 1970, the US Environmental Protection Agency (USEPA) has approved hundreds of thousands of chemicals for daily use; chemicals which leach into the soil, air, waterways, food – and breast milk (Steingraber, 2001). On the positive side, breastfeeding rates have continued to rise and, except in the most extreme cases, breast milk is *still* best, even as environmentalists strive to ban more and more toxins (Boswell-Penc, 2006).

Let's jump ahead now to Friday 14 June 2002. Again, imagine yourself sipping your morning tea and reading your paper. In June and July of that year, the Center for Children's Environmental Health, a research and advocacy group based at the Mount Sinai Hospital in New York, launched a consciousness-raising campaign that included a series of seven full-page warnings in the *New York Times*. Opening your paper, you will find a picture of a mother breastfeeding. The tag line reads: 'Our most precious natural resource is being threatened. Why?' The headings include the statements, 'Toxic chemicals are being passed on to infants in breast milk', and 'What We Can Do?' (Center for Children's Environmental Health, 2002). The campaign states in bold type that 'breastmilk is still best for mothers and children', but argues that this may not continue to be the case if we do not work to reverse course (Boswell-Penc, 2006). It urges us to pressure industries to use alternatives and governmental agencies to force compliance.

The very existence of this campaign means that by 2002 enough women were breastfeeding that scaring them into action might have some impact. The campaign continues today to raise people's awareness of the dangers of toxins, which I call 'level 2 environmental issues'; in many ways, these pale in comparison to what I refer to as 'level 1 environmental issues', that is, climate change and global depletion.

Full embodiment

Awareness of level 2 environmental issues help guide movement towards the kind of world we want to create and inhabit. It helps us when it comes to making choices between breast milk and formula, cow's milk and non-dairy alternatives. And it guides our responses to scenes of full embodiment versus scenes of disembodiment. If toxins are found in all mothers' milk, that should be a wake-up call. This is an environmental justice issue, an issue of privilege: racism, classism, sexism and ageism all play roles here, as more privileged women tend to live in places that render their breast milk healthier (Boswell-Penc, 2006); this knowledge can and should guide policy-making. At the same time, factory farming (and many other) industries participate in rendering mother's milk less and less 'fit for human consumption', since chemicals enter the food chain (Carson, 1962; Steingraber, 2001). Pesticides, petrochemicals, bovine growth hormones, antibiotics and other chemicals are used in growing feed grains, in the production of formula and in the dairy and meat industries (Boswell-Penc, 2006).

Non-dairy milk alternatives require much less resource-intensive production, and come with less intense level 2 environmental burdens, or toxins (Goodland and Anhang, 2009; Hertwich et al, 2010; Eshel et al, 2014). Soy, almond, coconut, rice and hemp milk involve lower body burdens of toxins, even when produced with pesticides and other chemicals, because they sit lower on the food chain than cow's milk. (Gartner, 2005; Foer, 2009; Oppenlander, 2012). Breast milk is better than infant formula in this regard because it provides more protection against a host of conditions (Steingraber, 2001; Boswell-Penc, 2006).

Human breast milk is associated with full embodiment not only because it involves the mother–child dyad, but because it requires no farmland, no pesticides, no petrochemicals, no CAFOs, no toxic run-off from sludge pools containing too much animal waste, and no machines for milking, pasteurising, packaging and transporting. Similar arguments can be made for non-dairy milk alternatives although these still require machines for pasteurising, packaging and transporting.

But what about level 1 environmental issues – climate change and global depletion? Several recent studies (Steinfeld, 2006; Goodland and Anhang, 2009; Hertwich et al, 2010) have highlighted the huge environmental impacts of the meat and dairy industries, as the climate change caused by these industries has an impact on everything from ocean acidification to waning biodiversity, species extinction and land use (Klein, 2014; Kolbert, 2014). A United Nations Food and Agriculture Organization (FAO) report, *Livestock's Long Shadow*, found that 18% of all global human-induced greenhouse gas emissions (GHG) come from the raising of animals for food (Steinfeld, 2006). Three years later, a World Bank study put that figure at 51% of annual GHG emissions (Goodland and Anhang, 2009). Somewhere between one fifth and one half of all greenhouse gas emissions come from livestock and dairy production. The United Nations has become so concerned that it has released a report suggesting a global shift towards a plant-based diet as a countermeasure (Hertwich et al, 2010). This position is supported by statistics on the differences in carbon output for various foods; indeed, the Environmental Working Group has published a study which lays out the full lifecycle of greenhouse gas emissions from common proteins and vegetables (Hamerschlag, 2011) (see Figure 2). In Figure 2 we see that consuming lamb generates the highest level of emissions, at 39.3 kg of CO_2 for every kilogram eaten, while consuming beef comes in second, generating 27.1 kg of CO_2 for each kilogram eaten (Environmental Working Group, 2007). Cheese consumption accounts for the third highest level of emissions, while consuming beans carries low emissions (Environmental Working Group, 2007). Low-fat milk and yoghurt sits low on the scale in terms of consumption, but full-fat milk and other dairy products sit high.

Today, many estimates concur that 30–50% of all GHG emissions come from raising animals for meat and dairy – including the production of milk for formula (Goodland and Anhang, 2009; Steinfeld, 2006). Giving babies breast milk followed by a plant-based diet does more to limit climate change than taking public transportation, driving an electric car or riding a bicycle, although these are all great ways to reduce carbon emissions as well (Goodland and Anhang, 2009;

Figure 2: Full lifecycle of greenhouse gas emissions from common proteins and vegetables

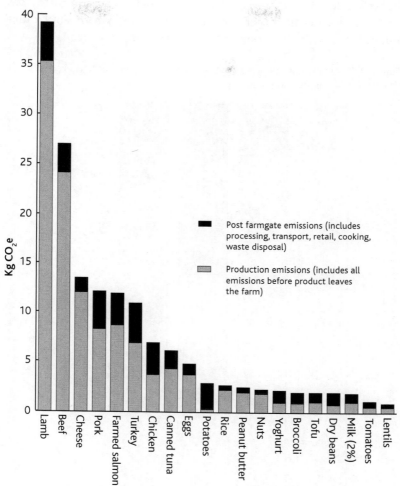

Source: © Environmental Working Group (2011) Reproduced with permission.

Simon, 2013). Why? Because ruminants produce methane gas, which is approximately 25 times more potent than carbon dioxide in contributing to climate change (Goodland and Anhang, 2009; Simon, 2013). Cows are the most populous ruminant on Earth owing to meat and dairy production. It is estimated that 75% of global arable land is used for grazing and 'sheltering' animals for meat and dairy, and for producing cereal grains for animal feed (Simon, 2013). Figure 3 presents a table from the Proceedings of the National Academy of Scientists of the United States of America (Eshel et al, 2014). This shows the percentage of the overall national environmental burdens exerted by individual animal categories. While these figures pertain to the US, one can surmise that other industrialised countries with similar diets might have similar environmental burdens.

Figure 3: Percentage of the overall national environmental burdens exerted by the individual animal categories

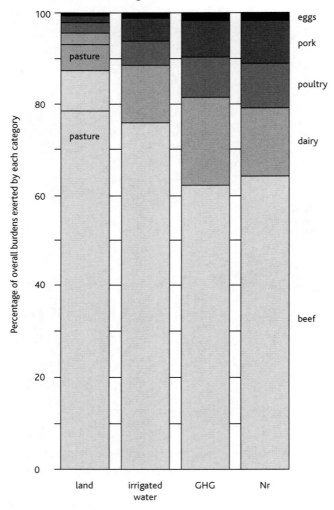

Source: Eshel et al (2014). © National Academy of Sciences. Reproduced with permission.

The authors say that:

> The results are obtained by multiplying the values of Fig.
> 2E, recast as annual overall national caloric consumption, by
> the resource per megacalorie of Fig. 2 A–D. Beef requires
> ≈88% of all US land allocated to producing animal-based
> calories, partitioned (from the bottom up) among pasture
> (≈79%), processed roughage (≈7%), and concentrated feed
> (≈2%). The land demands of dairy are displayed in the same
> format. (Nr refers to reactive nitrogen burdens). (Eshel et
> al, 2014: 11998)

Rainforests house the greatest biological diversity on Earth and provide the greatest source of carbon offsets (Eschel et al, 2014). We destroy rainforests to grow cereals for animal food, or we use the cleared land for grazing (Foer, 2009; Eschel et al, 2014). According to the Intergovernmental Panel on Climate Change (IPCC), 75% of all the land that is used for pasturing animals and for growing animal feed is in the process of being turned into desert (IPCC, 2014). Fertile topsoil is a precious, vital resource, but it is being eroded and/or depleted by being used to produce feed grains for billions of animals – animals that are intensively confined, force-fed and slaughtered at a fraction of their full lifespan (Foer, 2009; Goodland and Anhang 2009; Oppenlander, 2012). This process of land management and animal processing is simply not sustainable and not compassionate.

As Nibert points out, 'No other sector of the capitalist system is endangering the Earth and all its inhabitants more than the animal industrial complex' (Nibert, 2013). Indeed, a 2008 report issued by the US National Intelligence Council warned that expansion of the Western diet and climate change will 'yield a tangle of difficult to manage consequences' by 2030 (NIC, 2008: 52). A 2008 report by senior European Union officials warned that 'increased competition for water, grain and energy ha[s] the potential to create significant conflicts in Africa, the Middle East and between Russia and the European Union' (quoted in Nibert, 2013).

While we have long known that formula production weighs quite heavily in resource use compared to breast milk, we are just starting to recognise the differences between resource use in meat-and-dairy versus plant based diets. If we look briefly at the number of calories of fossil fuel energy that it takes to produce meat, as opposed to plant-based foods, the numbers are significant (Chrispeels and Sadava, 1994;

Steinfeld et al, 2006). This is particularly pronounced when we consider projections for increases in human population.

Climate-changing gases are released in the production of foods that have the potential to make our bodies significantly less healthy. Indeed, growing evidence points to links – some showing correlations, others pointing to causation – between the consumption of meat and dairy, and rising obesity rates, as well as rising incidence of diabetes; cardiovascular disease; arterial hypertension; breast, prostrate, ovarian and colon cancers; spectrum disorders including attention deficit disorder; Alzheimer's; dementia; fibromyalgia and Crohn's disease (Fuhrman, 2003; Ornish, 2003; Campbell and Campbell, 2005; Tuttle, 2005; Oppenlander, 2012).

Much has been written on the 'omnivore's dilemma'– Michael Pollan's title – which posits a diet including meat and dairy, but only that which has been produced organically on small, responsibly managed farms (Pollan, 2006). While much can be said on this, animals raised in a 'responsible' way are indeed better for our environment and our bodies, and at the same time, in terms of sustaining Earth's resources, the less meat and dairy we consume, the better (Goodland and Anhang, 2009; Eshel et al, 2014). We can add to this the fact that as the consequences of climate change on the Earth and on human societies intensify, other public health issues will also intensify (Foer 2009; Goodland and Anhang, 2009), including diseases from insect vectors, food insecurity owing to farmland flooding, water insecurity and increasing drought, and strife between host communities and roaming environmental refugees (Oppenlander, 2012; Klein, 2014).

Embodiment as compassion

So far, I have focused primarily on differences in health outcomes, environmental effects and resource use in contrasting breast milk and infant formula, and cow's milk and non-dairy alternatives. But also at stake are less tangible differences such as the relationship between compassion and embodiment. Different degrees of embodiment involve subtle, or not-so-subtle, effects on babies, children and mothers, but also on cows and calves, indeed, on planet Earth, and all the diverse ecosystems that make up our home. Speciesism emerges as a necessary consideration if we are to take full stock of this impasse at which we, as a global community, currently reside. The assumption that only our own species deserves to be taken into consideration as we make far-reaching decisions about life, death, health and survival seems hubristic at best and exceedingly dangerous at worst. Our arrival at this point, where human health and ecosystem health are at stake, points to the limits of our understanding. Placing ourselves at the centre of decision-making about Earth's resources has shown itself to be not only unhealthy but unsustainable. It leads not only to resource depletion and climate change, but also to a dwindling of the Earth's biodiversity, a grave danger for the long-term survival of our planet (Kolbert, 2014). Some have also argued that a consequence of speciesism is that our self-centred approach weighs heavily on our psyches and, as a result, renders us less compassionate, less evolved and less fulfilled than we could be (Tuttle, 2005; Harper, 2010; Oppenlander, 2012).

The choices we face between mother's milk and formula for babies, and cow's milk and non-dairy alternatives for children and adults, invite us to look at possibilities for creating worlds very different from the one we currently inhabit. Breastfeeding advocates have long argued that profound differences in children's and mothers' health emerge when we compare breast milk and formula (Carson, 1962; Steingraber, 2001; Boswell-Penc, 2006). These include psychosocial and cognitive differences (Steingraber, 2001; Boswell-Penc, 2006).

Similarly, some have argued that plant-based diets offer psychosocial and cognitive benefits (Tuttle, 2005; Harper, 2010; Oppenlander, 2012). They point to the violence, misery and brutality of our industrial farming systems, and to the ways in which:

> confining and killing animals for food … brings violence into our bodies and minds and disturbs the physical, emotional, mental, social and spiritual dimensions of ourselves in deep and intractable ways. (Tuttle, 2005: 10)

A world with dairy produced in an industrialised farming system is a world with beef and veal. Here, female calves are subjected to the same brutal lives as their mothers (Webster, 1986; Scully, 2002; Tuttle, 2005; Oppenlander, 2012). Males, on the other hand, become essential components in the veal and beef industries, and thus become the central inextricable link which connects the meat and dairy industries in an industrial complex.

In the industrialised farming system which is characteristic of the US, UK and other similarly industrialised countries, cows are subjected to intensive practices which drastically affect the quality of their lives. Repeated and ongoing artificial insemination allows lactation to be controlled and managed on efficiency/economic grounds (Webster, 1986). Cows are denied access to their young and given pharmaceutical products which cause adverse side effects and bring about other diseases, and problems such as lameness and mastitis (Webster, 1986; USDA, 2007; Drugs.com, 2014). Embodiment is key here. When we are disembodied, we lack presence (Tuttle, 2005). By feeding into the churning of habitual messages telling us to speed up, consume more, opt for the most convenient options, we not only lack presence, we lack compassion (Tuttle, 2005; Harper, 2010; Oppenlander, 2012). When we are disembodied, we stop being in touch with the best choices, the healthiest paths, the most wholesome, nutrient-rich foods, and the ways of living that are best for us and Planet Earth. Coming into presence, perhaps while breastfeeding our child, has the potential to change everything.

When we come into mindfulness, we start to sense the best options. We see that it is best to breastfeed our babies and children, and if possible to do so for an extended period. We see that the second best option is to use a breast pump or express breast milk by hand, even if we 'feel like a cow'. Or, facing difficulties, we might opt for milk from a human milk bank. We might begin to have compassion for ourselves, and for the cows, those gentle, intelligent, loving creatures who deserve to suckle their own calves and not be subjected to lives of pain and deprivation. And we might see that while not all dairy products, beef and meat come out of an intensive industrial farming system, all dairy products, meat and infant formula production does burden our ecosystem with methane and resource use that exacerbates climate change and places greater strain on our Earth, pushing us closer to the limits of the planet's carrying capacity.

Conclusion

It is telling that differing degrees of embodiment can be seen to correspond with various stages of human interaction with the Earth. As scientific historian Carolyn Merchant points out, the science associated with the Industrial Revolution can be seen to correlate with the historical phase that viewed Earth as inert; this model increasingly saw infant formula as being 'as good as' mother's milk (Merchant, 1989). But the evolution of science has also brought us to more complex understandings which help us to better understand human and ecosystem health.

This science, more holistic, more embodied and also more 'compassionate', has the potential to show us the perils of choosing food production and consumption patterns that come from a disregard for human and ecosystem health (Gartner, 2005; Goodland and Anhang, 2009; Oppenlander, 2012). This science, more willing to disregard assumptions of a split between the 'subjective' and the 'objective', has the potential to help us realise that we have choices; we can work together to bring embodiment to the fore as a guide to optimal health for all. Research indicates that we make healthier decisions when we focus on others as well as ourselves (Poulin et al, 2013). Considering full embodiment as a key component for achieving individual, public and planetary health has the potential to help breastfeeding professionals make a case for exclusive and extended breastfeeding.

References

American Diabetic Association (2003) 'Position of the American Diabetic Association and dieticians of Canada: vegetarian diets', *Journal of American Diabetic Association*, 103: 748–65.

Boswell-Penc (2006) *Tainted milk: Breastmilk, feminisms and the politics of environmental degradation*, Albany, NY: SUNY Press.

Boswell-Penc, M. and Boyer, K. (2007) '"Expressing anxiety?" Breast pump usage in American wage workplaces', *Gender Place and Culture*, 14 (5): 551–67.

Campbell, T. C. and Campbell, T. M. (2005) *The China study: The most comprehensive study of nutrition ever conducted and the startling implications for diet, weight loss and long-term health*, Dallas, TX: BenBella Books.

Carson, R. (1962) *Silent spring*, Boston, MA: Houghton Mifflin.

Center for Children's Environmental Health (2002) 'Our most precious resource is being threatened. Why?', *New York Times*, June 14: Section A.

Chrispeels, M. J. and Sadava, D. E. (1994) *Plants, genes and crop biotechnology*, Sudbury, MA: Jones and Bartlett Publishers.

Dobson, B. and Murtaugh, A. (2001) 'Position of the American Dietetic Association: Breaking the barriers to breastfeeding', *Journal of the Academy of Nutrition and Dietetics*, 101(10): 1213–20.

Drugs.com (2014) 'Treatments for dairy cattle', www.drugs.com/vet/dairy-cattle-a.html

Environmental Defense Fund, (2002) 'Where it all began', www.environmentaldefense.org/

Environmental Working Group (2007) 'Meat eaters guide to climate change: Full life cycle of greenhouse gas emissions from common proteins and vegetables', www.ewg.org

Environmental Working Group (2011) 'Eat smart. Your food choices affect the climate', www.ewg.org/meateatersguide/eat-smart/

Eshel, G., Shepon, A., Makov, T. and Milo, R. (2014) 'Land, irrigation water, greenhouse gas, and reactive nitrogen burdens of meat, eggs, and dairy production in the United States', *Proceedings of the National Academy of Sciences*, 111: 11996–12001.

Foer, J. (2009) *Eating animals*, New York, NY: Back Bay Books.

Fuhrman, J. (2003) *Eat to live: The revolutionary formula for fast and sustainable weight loss*, New York, NY: Little Brown and Company.

Gartner, L. M. (2005) 'Breastfeeding and the use of human milk', *Pediatrics*, 115(2): 496–506.

Goldman, A. S. (2000) 'Modulation of the gastrointestinal tract of infants by human milk, interfaces and interactions: an evolutionary perspective', *Journal of Nutrition*, 130: 426s–31s.

Goodland, R. and Anhang, J. (2009) 'Livestock and climate change: what if the key actors in climate change are... cows, pigs, and chickens?', *World Watch Institute Magazine*, 22(6): 10–19.

Grossman, E. (2014) 'As dairy farms grow bigger, new concerns about pollution', *Yale Environment*, 360, http://e360.yale.edu/features/as_dairy_farms_grow_bigger_new_concerns_about_pollution

Hamerschlag, K. (2011) 'What you eat matters', Environmental Working Group, www.ewg.org/meateatersguide

Harper, A. B. (2010) *Sistah vegan: Black female vegans speak on food, identity, health and society*, New York: Lantern Books.

Hertwich, E., Van der Voet, E., Suh, S., Tukker, A., Huijbregts, M., Kazmierczyk, P., Lenzen, M., McNeely, J. and Moriguchi, Y. (2010) 'Assessing the environmental impacts of consumption and production: Priority products and materials: a report of the working group on the environmental impacts of products and materials to the international panel for sustainable resource management', United Nations Environment Programme, www.unep.org/publications

Host, A. (2002) 'Frequency of cow's milk allergy in childhood', *Annals of Allergy, Asthma and Immunology*, 89 (6, S1): 33–7.

IPCC (2014) 'Climate change 2014: Synthesis report: Contribution of working groups I, II and III to the fifth assessment report of the Intergovernmental Panel on Climate Change', Geneva, Switzerland: IPCC.

Klein, N. (2014) *This changes everything: Capitalism vs. the climate*, New York, NY: Simon and Schuster.

Kolbert, E. (2014) *The sixth great extinction: An unnatural history*, New York, NY: Henry Holt and Company.

Ludington-Hoe, S. and Swinth, J. Y. (1996) 'Developmental aspects of kangaroo care', *Journal of Obstetric, Gynocologic, and Neonatal Nursing*, 25: 691–703.

Mayo Clinic (2016) 'Infant formula: your questions answered', Mayo Clinic, www.mayoclinic.org/healthy-lifestyle/infant-and-toddler-health/in-depth/infant-formula/art-20045782

Merchant, C. (1989) *The death of nature: Women, ecology and the scientific revolution*, San Francisco, CA: Harper and Row.

National Intelligence Council (2008) 'Global trends 2025: A transformed world', www.foresightfordevelopment.org/sobipro/55/758-global-trends-2025-a-transformed-world

Nibert, D. (2013) 'The animal industrial complex', Cleveland, OH: Alternative Radio, https://www.alternativeradio.org/products/nibd001#

Oppenlander, R. A. (2012) *Comfortably unaware: What we choose to eat is killing us and our planet*, New York, NY: Beaufort Books.

Ornish, D. (2003) 'The killer American diet that's sweeping the planet', https://www.ted.com/talks/dean_ornish_on_the_world_s_killer_diet

Pollan, M. (2006) *The omnivore's dilemma*, New York: The Gale Group.

Poulin M. J., Brown S. L., Dillard A. J. and Smith D. M. (2013) 'Giving to others and the association between stress and mortality', American *Journal of Public Health*, 103: 1649–55.

Rollins, N. C, Bhandari, N., Hajeebhoy, N., Horton, S., Lutter, C. K., Martines, J. C., Piwoz, E. G., Richter, L. M., and Victora, C. G., on behalf of The Lancet Breastfeeding Series Group (2016) 'Why invest, and what it will take to improve breastfeeding practices?', *Lancet*, 387(10017): 491–504.

Rowe, M. (ed) (1999) *The way of compassion: Vegetarianism, environmentalism, animal advocacy and social justice*, New York: Stealth Technologies.

Scariati, P., Grummer-Strawn, L. and Fein, S. (1997) 'A longitudinal analysis of infant morbidity and the extent of breastfeeding in the United States', *Pediatrics*, 9(6): e5.

Scully, M. (2002) *Dominion: The power of man, the suffering of animals, and the call to mercy*, New York: St. Martin's Griffin.

Simon, D. R. (2013) 'The Meatanomics index', https://meatonomics.com/2013/08/22/meatonomics-index

Steinfeld, H. (2006) *Livestock's long shadow: Environmental issues and options*, Rome: Food and Agriculture Organization of the United Nations.

Steingraber, S. (2001) *Having faith: An ecologist's journey to motherhood*, Cambridge: Perseus Publishing.

Tuttle, W. (2005) *The world peace diet: Eating for spiritual health and social harmony*, New York: Lantern Books.

USDA (2007) 'Animal health', www.aphis.usda.gov/animal_health/nahms/dairy/downloads/dairy07/Dairy07_is_ReprodPrac.pdf

Victora, C. G., Bahl, R., Barros, A.J.D., Franca, G.V.A., Horton, S., Krasevec, J., Murch, S., Sankar, M. J., Walker, N. and Rollins, N. C., on behalf of the Lancet Breastfeeding Series Group (2016) 'Breastfeeding in the 21st century: epidemiology, mechanisms, and lifelong effect', *Lancet*, 387(10017): 403–504.

Weber, K. (ed) (2009) *Food, Inc.: How industrial food is making us sicker, fatter and poorer – and what you can do about it*, New York, NY: Participant Media.

Webster J. (1986) 'Health and welfare of animals in modern husbandry systems: dairy cattle', *In Practice*, May 8(3): 85–9.

Wuethrich, B. (2003) 'Infectious disease: chasing the fickle swine flu', *Science*, 299: 1502–5.

Yale University (2001) 'Animal-based nutrients linked with higher risk of stomach and esophageal cancers', news release, 15 October, http://news.yale.edu/2001/10/15/animal-based-nutrients-linked-higher-risk-stomach-and-esophageal-cancers

Breastfeeding and popular culture: reflections for policy and practice

Nicki Symes, Elizabeth Mayo and Emma Laird

Introduction

This commentary is informed by personal written reflections as well as ideas from a conversation, both of which sparked our engagement with the chapters and the meaning of the seminar series to us. Quotes within the chapter are from these conversations and reflections; we decided not to identify ourselves in relation to these.

Something about us

We each came to the seminar series with different experiences of society, as women, mothers and workers. Between us, in our personal and professional lives and over 30 years, we have lived through many phases of infant feeding policy and practice. Early and late maternity is part of our experience:

> 'I have had four children over 23 years, I became a mum at the age of 18 and had my last baby when I was 40 years old, which has taken me on my breastfeeding journey. I have also become a grandparent, so I have been able to support my daughter and her partner at the beginning of their journey as parents.'

The seminars gave us time to reflect on breastfeeding in a group setting with some novel and fresh approaches, as well as more familiar ones. Women breastfeed in a social context, and one thing that struck us about the series was that it was about sharing women's stories. This prompted us to share ours a little:

> 'I realise that I was lucky to have far fewer obstacles in my way when breastfeeding my girls. The majority of women in my wider community breastfed; I had an encouraging and supportive partner and great care. I was breastfed during

the '60s — I remember my mum being really proud of this — and my grandmothers breastfed a total of 11 babies in the 1930s and '40s!'

The seminars brought home the different stories of women who must navigate complex societal and cultural barriers to start and keep breastfeeding. The three of us support them in different ways, covering the voluntary sector, public health and early years services, providing support for women, leadership, national and local strategy development, and commissioning services. Our common desire is to improve the experience for breastfeeding women; we have seen shifting professional practice over time and we want all women to have what they need:

'Over the years there have been changes to the way mothers are informed of things. I still feel there needs to be many more changes to empower parents and support them.'

Each one of us has been involved in the Unicef UK Baby Friendly Initiative, either directly or indirectly, and seen how training transforms individuals' views; each small step a move towards cultural change.

So, have the seminars changed how we perceive breastfeeding?

'As a public health practitioner/commissioner, I valued the seminars. They have offered a time to pause, reflect and think about the bigger picture, to meet with others to consider some of the wider theoretical perspectives, policy and ideas.'

'As a practitioner, I was able to have a free space which was good, as budgets are tight in many services. It provided me with a great opportunity to meet other professionals with many different backgrounds to myself. As I work for a children's centre, I was able to talk with others about the work I do, and how I feel we can make changes. It was also interesting to listen to the guest speakers from around the world, and have table discussions. Many different views were shared and valued, which was a positive experience.'

The public/private division of breastfeeding

Perhaps the public/private division of breastfeeding isn't so relevant these days, when mothers have easy access to social media. Their brelfies are statements that invite us into their world, and redefine these aspects of breastfeeding. Giles's chapter (Chapter Ten) helps us reimagine what breastfeeding 'in public' really means, by distinguishing between solitary and social breastfeeding. Solitary is 'private' between the mother and baby only; they may be hidden away in a breastfeeding room while out and about. Social breastfeeding, on the other hand, is when others are around; this may be in the mother's house, in shared social spaces at the table or at work (Giles, Chapter Ten). Fraser (Chapter Nine) points out, though, that UK work practices may push mothers to wean and, as Giles notes, may deny 'breastfeeding its rightful place within the social' (Chapter Ten: 189).

Brelfies are powerful. They are mothers dismantling the solitary/social and making breastfeeding social. Their selfies reach a wide audience and invite onlookers in. We might think about how this makes onlookers feel. Some mothers fear negative comments when breastfeeding outside the home; however, brelfies don't appear to attract negative responses online. Does this make it safer for mothers? How may they develop resilience strategies?

Mothers drive this new view of breastfeeding – so is it rebellion when mothers pose with napkins on their heads when asked to cover up? Does it set new expectations that mothers should post their brelfies? Would others' brelfies help pregnant women make the shift and increase self-efficacy? It raised lots of issues for us:

> 'It may be part of their journey; it can be positive to share these things. By seeing the photos we may be missing mums who are struggling, who are hiding behind their smiling brelfies.'

How far will these women get without wider society also assuming its role? Practitioners are familiar with the Unicef Call to Action (2016). Mothers are changing the conversation themselves to socially integrated breastfeeding, however policy should adapt and empower mothers to continue breastfeeding. This will take political will. We need political will to take responsibility for removing barriers, which can then open doors to breastfeeding: by recognising that giving a woman time antenatally to visit a breastfeeding support group should be part of her NHS care, and by including the value of breast milk in the UK's gross national product and protecting working rights for mothers who return to paid work while breastfeeding.

Images of breasts

Altering breastfeeding imagery by shifting the perception of breasts from sexual to maternal is essential for change (Giles, Chapter Ten) so that the normalisation of breastfeeding can happen (Bartlett, Chapter Eleven). Seeing breastfeeding affects womens' feeding decisions. So how can we use this in our work? By encouraging mothers to meet up and share and record their stories to inspire others, helping them to see that they are not alone. Seeing breastfeeding can evoke strong feelings, and practitioners may help women explore those feelings.

Imagery from the public world of art, or the domestic domain via brelfies, is augmented by other examples of empowered use of space when breastfeeding. MPs in Iceland and Australia have addressed their parliaments while breastfeeding – a great example of empowerment (see, for example, England, 2016; BBC News, 2017).Representational art may help empower women through interaction with everyday images as well as images like Skywhale. Hearing about Skywhale was fascinating. Through it we can engage with lactational breast imagery in a unique, creative, playful and empowering way, although the 'cow-like' imagery could perhaps put some women off. An alternative image of the everyday in relation to breastfeeding could be Benjamin Sullivan's 2017 BP Portrait Award-winning painting of a woman sitting on a chair in her dressing gown breastfeeding her baby daughter. Breastfeeding photographs can be used antenatally to help women and partners address their emotions. Including a picture of Skywhale among these may even heighten those responses, but that may not be a negative thing. Working through their emotions, with our support 'holding' them in a safe place, may increase mothers' self-efficacy.

Breastfeeding and the ecological precipice

Breastfeeding is the most effective form of nutrition for our babies. It also links us to all humankind (Bartlett, Chapter Eleven). This is important because 'as we reside at a precipice in terms of public health … Breast milk for young ones and non-dairy milk for others emerges as critical to securing optimal health for all' (Boswell-Penc, Chapter Twelve: 219).

Boswell-Penc itemises the societal resources needed to produce infant formula. She makes the connection between industrialised dairy farms and mothers who express milk. Releasing mothers to fully breastfeed leads to better health and diet for babies – and our planet. How do we share this? Social context is important: the 1970s US information campaign she discusses rebounded. Practitioners know that breastfeeding promotion messages are nuanced and don't always lend themselves well to portrayal in the media. As Boswell-Penc notes in Chapter Twelve, the reworded 2002 campaign in the US took place when breastfeeding rates were higher, and it was better received. Practitioners are aware that national breastfeeding campaigns don't necessarily shift breastfeeding rates. It will be interesting to see whether social media campaigns like the English 'Breastfeeding Celebration Week' make a difference to future initiation and maintenance rates, and whether brelfies affect breastfeeding promotion. Presenting information such as that discussed in Chapter Ten can be seen as affecting breastfeeding promotion. Practitioners might consider whether their role includes promoting breastfeeding, or protecting and supporting breastfeeding, or all three aspects.

Embodiment and empowerment

Embodiment and empowerment seem to fit with responsive breastfeeding. Breastfeeding is not just about food, but about meeting peoples' emotional and social needs. For some women, returning to work and expressing breast milk feels like being a cow. They feel disconnected from their bodies and are not with their babies. Supporters often suggest that a mother becomes tuned into what helps her to release oxytocin. For many mothers, it is using their senses – for example, having a recording of their baby on their phone or putting an item of their baby's clothing over their shoulder. Work barriers might exclude babies from workplaces to feed, which highlights the structural reforms needed to protect mothers' right to breastfeed through employment law (Fraser, Chapter Nine; Giles, Chapter Ten).

Breastfeeding, work and the law

A mulifaceted breastfeeding strategy needs individual countries to legislate and implement practices that support breastfeeding, such as adequate maternity pay/leave; it is in everyone's interest if breastfeeding rates rise. Norwegian mothers receive full salary for 10 months, or 80% salary for 12 months postnatally. Women public sector workers in Norway, for example, are entitled to two hours of paid breastfeeding breaks everyday, which they can take at the workplace or use to visit their child (Nordic Page, 2013). UK maternity leave and pay are less generous, and women's return to work after having a baby largely depends on their financial situation, as well as local arrangements.

Women need flexibility of approach and individualised planning. As a society, we need to reimagine work to allow more homeworking/ shorter days, phased returns and paid breastfeeding breaks.

Returning to work and leaving your baby for the first time can be very emotional, and mothers have to discuss how they will maintain lactation – requiring them to talk about bodily substances (Dowling, Chapter Three) – as well as navigate hierarchical structures. Managers are part of the wider community. They may have encountered grief, suffering or anger, for themselves or others, about not breastfeeding in a society that doesn't support breastfeeding. Fraser (Chapter Nine) outlines the law around workplace breastfeeding support and highlights what is needed to help this support to be available. We have experienced/witnessed some supportive practices:

> 'I have experienced examples of support that enables breastfeeding: lunchtime feeds of a baby brought to work by his father or the flexibility of ad hoc work, allowing short shifts to enable continued breastfeeding of an older baby.'

> 'My manager wasn't aware of a risk assessment for a nursing mother; he would be interested in seeing one so we can put this in place. I wasn't asked whether I wanted to express or store my milk. I think this is because I am aware of where I can store milk, but it was suggested that I could have my baby brought to me to feed. Instead, it was agreed that I could have a set lunch break and pop home to do this. I was told, "If you are tired or need a break just say and you can rest." I am taking a slow return to work.'

Such examples of good practice are heartening; sharing experience can help to create a culture in which breastfeeding is a real option. Making changes to practice can make a difference.

> 'I made sure that the "Welcome to Breastfeed" sign was in the right place and nursery staff now ask, "How is your baby being fed?"' We have welcome stickers on all of the buildings and a comfy stool or a chair in each corridor for breastfeeding. If mums need a quiet space we make this possible for them.'

Conclusion

So where do we go from here? The seminar series was a special time. It gave us information and insights into things we had never seen or thought about before. We met people from different parts of the country/world doing different jobs to us. What we all had in common was a desire to help women breastfeed their babies. As we wrote this commentary, we were able to identify things that we can take back into our everyday work, even from the more unusual presentations such as those on brelfies and Skywhale. Small things can have big consequences.

We've learnt that women are themselves changing the conversation around breastfeeding – however, societal change needs to shore that up. Public and health policy needs to take responsibility for changing the feeding culture, and put policies in place that enable mothers to breastfeed for as long as they want to. Breastfeeding is everybody's business.

References

BBC News (2017) 'Australian politician becomes first to breastfeed in parliament', *BBC News*, www.bbc.co.uk/news/world-australia-39853360

England, C. (2016) 'Icelandic MP breastfeeds baby during a debate in parliament', *Independent*, www.independent.co.uk/news/people/icelandic-mp-breastfeeds-baby-debate-parliament-al-ingi-a7358681.html

Nordic Page (2013) 'All Norwegian women to be paid for breastfeeding breaks', *Nordic Page*, https://www.tnp.no/norway/panorama/3586-all-norwegian-women-to-be-paid-for-breastfeeding-breaks

Unicef (2016) 'Call to action on infant feeding in the UK', Unicef, https://www.unicef.org.uk/babyfriendly/baby-friendly-resources/advocacy/call-to-action

Series context: reflection on experiences of attending the seminar series

Sally Tedstone

Attending the seminar series was a unique experience in which a range of participants from the fields of academia, practice and policy were brought together with the intention of creating the opportunity for 'collaborative knowledge creation'. I was interested to explore the extent to which the vehicle of the seminar series fulfilled this ambition and how the seminars were experienced by the range of attendees. In this short chapter I will share what I have discovered.

First, let's consider why bringing people together from different perspectives might be worthwhile. What do we imagine the value of collaborative knowledge creation would be? Since the early 1990s, an evidence-based medical approach to healthcare provision has been advocating for the greater use of research in clinical practice (De Brún, 2013). Evidence-based practice is seen as a marker of good-quality, effective health services, and is increasingly valued in the voluntary world too (Breastfeeding Network, 2016; NCT, 2017).

Alongside this, there has been a parallel move towards evidence-based policy (Parliament UK, 2011) which supports giving significant weight to research evidence as policies are shaped. In addition, academics who carry out this research are increasingly aware of the importance of being able to demonstrate 'user value', and the impact of research on the economy and society, which in the UK is reported via the Research Excellence Framework (Research Excellence Framework, 2014). However, embedding research into practice and policy in a meaningful way presents many challenges. As practitioners the evidence about the things that challenge us is not necessarily available to us and it sometimes seems that nobody is studying the things we have questions about. Policy makers are not always aware of the research that could inform policy. Researchers don't always understand what practitioners or policy makers struggle with, or do not have funding to study these areas. Buse et al (2005) use the concept of two communities (university researchers and government officials) to describe this set of challenges. This seminar series started from the premise of three communities: academics, policy makers and practitioners. There appears to be a consensus that there is a need for more dialogue and closer working. Practical steps advocated by Buse et al include conferences, seminars and workshops to disseminate research findings. The seminar series on which this book draws is an example of such an endeavour. Careful thought was given to the organisation of each seminar to maximise the likelihood of meaningful dialogue. There was purposeful mixing of participants on tables to avoid people sitting in peer groups. Plenty of time was allowed for discussion of the presentations. This gave the event a less formal atmosphere: it felt to me less like, 'Here we all are to sit and listen to these clever people and learn,' and more like, 'This is interesting. What do we all, from our different viewpoints, think about this and how can this help us?'

Feedback from the final seminar was very positive. Without exception, the events had been enjoyable and interesting for all categories of participants. So, the series was successful on one level, but beyond this, to what extent was there evidence that the goal of collaborative knowledge creation had been achieved? What would this look like? On the one hand, this could be tangible knowledge products such as joint publications, the development of ideas for new research questions, and joint research proposals and projects. Alongside this, I would suggest that there is another dimension including awareness and developing an understanding of others' perspectives on issues. This is a softer outcome, difficult to measure but nonetheless important. Reviewing the feedback at the end of the series, with these softer outcomes in mind, I found many examples. There was a strong sense that practitioners felt 'nourished' and 'buoyed up'. This is worthwhile; often in practice settings there is little time for learning, discussion and reflection. In addition, several practitioners were keen to look for opportunities to be involved in research. Practitioners as part of research teams are an asset, bringing the two 'communities' together with a tangible impact on outcomes. For example, research proposals will be developed with an inbuilt reality check, and better communication between research teams and practitioners will mean that projects are more likely to meet recruitment targets and interventions are more likely to be implemented as intended.

Academics valued being able to sense-check their work 'in the real world' and the opportunity to understand more about the challenges facing practitioners. They were also looking forward to working on collaborative projects. Policy makers were not well represented in the series. Those that attended valued the opportunity to link more closely with researchers and were keen to bring the learning from the seminar into service development, although no concrete plans were evident at the time of writing.

A core group of participants were able to attend the majority of the sessions and were perhaps best placed to realise the goal of creative knowledge creation. When preparing this chapter, I asked the core group to share their reflections. Academics reported that they found the series both useful and challenging. Lisa said:

'This series felt quite different to attending academic seminars, where everyone is focused on academic rather than policy or practice questions. While the atmosphere was very friendly and open, I did find it quite challenging to have to put academic ideas to work in conversations with practitioners and policy makers, who have a much more "hands-on" approach to the everyday challenges and realities of breastfeeding promotion.'

Melanie reported that she valued an audience who understood her, and continued:

'I enjoyed the chance to be able to speak without having to lay extensive foundations first, and to simply state my argument without having to prepare the way.'

Her feedback also demonstrated evidence of the value of being able to understand the world of the practitioners:

'I found it very valuable to be with people from different viewpoints in terms of their role in working with breastfeeding women. Those working on the ground have a particularly challenging role, as they have to synthesise research, policy, information and how to support an emotional (often distraught) woman. Hearing how they do this, especially in situations where resources are so constrained, is incredibly valuable for me and informs my practice as an academic. I want to do research which is useful and has impact. Therefore, I need to hear these stories.'

The way the seminars were run seemed to be successful. The small table work, in particular, was commented on by Dawn:

'These small groups were important ... not just for broadening understanding, but also for increasing engagement with others from a different background. We often hear about the importance of dialogue between academics, practitioners and policy makers but it's easy for people to be silenced in a meeting by thinking, "I'm out of touch with practice/the real world," or, "I'm not academic enough," or, "I can't actually remember what BFI says about x, y or z." In small groups people could more happily share their perceived ignorance and learn from each other! So, if this doesn't sound too cheesy, I'm talking about the importance of understanding the social experience not just of breastfeeding, but also the social experience of building bridges between research, policy and practice.'

Non-academics in the core group found the series enjoyable and stimulating, but had some comments on accessibility, particularly concerning language. As Nicki commented, "At times I think some of the presentations were presented in less accessible language." I am aware that the seminar series organisers worked hard with the presenters to support them in their use of accessible language. This was clearly essential although not always accomplished.

The seminar series organisers were also asked share their reflections on the series, and these were rich and honest. They were pleased to have achieved many of the things they set out to do, these were: to include a range of academics (some international); to cover a breadth of topics and achieve a broad perspective; to create opportunities to involve early career researchers and finally; to reach out to an audience of academics, practitioners and policy makers. They recognised and valued highly the ethos of inclusivity that they had created. The core group was created to allow relationships to build over time and provide an important link between each individual seminar, with a sense of the series building over the two years. However, they were disappointed that conversations between each seminar were not easy to foster.

Reflecting on the extent to which the academics were able to adjust their language to that appropriate for the mixed audience of the series, David commented, "Some people were just not able to do it." One aspect which the organisers felt they could have worked harder at was reaching out to practitioners and making it easier for them to attend.

One very interesting outcome of the series, for me personally, has been the conversations I have had with other core group members, in order to write the chapter commentaries. This has been a useful way to ensure that our aspirations to use the ideas and conversations stimulated by the series are taken further. Making time for these 'beyond the seminar series' conversations has been tricky, and to be honest, probably would not have happened for me without my commitment to develop these reflective chapters.

Overall, it is clear that the series was enjoyable and valued by the participants, and that there is some evidence, even at this relatively early stage, that the aim of collaborative knowledge creation was achieved. At the time of writing, there are some 'knowledge products' in development, mostly in the form of articles and book chapters. There are also some ideas of how things could be done differently that are being explored, for example, my approach to infant feeding updates for practitioners (in my role as Infant Feeding Lead in local maternity services) has become broader, more reflective and inclusive of social science research, and this seems popular. What is also clear to me, however, is that a seminar series, while an extremely good idea, is not in itself enough to ensure that the goal of truly collaborative knowledge creation is achieved. Everyone is busy; it is hard to find the time, space and energy to explore new ideas or ways of working – and yet, it is vital that we do. Mechanisms to support the continued exploration of ideas conceived at the seminars are essential if they are to bear fruit. Collaborating on a book or a follow-up seminar presentation stimulates progress. If there was funding for small pilot projects following on from the series, there would be a real incentive to take the seeds of ideas that started to germinate and nurture them to fruitfulness. I will finish with the thoughts again of Dawn, one of the core group members:

> 'I think it's up to us to make it useful though. I can sit in my office and forget all about the work of the people I met or I can look up their work and keep in contact and maybe develop further collaboration.'

References

Breastfeeding Network (2016) 'Our vision and aims', https://www.breastfeedingnetwork.org.uk/charitable-objectives

Buse, K., Mays, N. and Walt, G. (2005) *Making health policy*, Maidenhead: Open University Press.

De Brún, C. (2013) 'Finding the evidence: A key step in the information production process', https://www.england.nhs.uk/wp-content/uploads/2017/02/tis-guide-finding-the-evidence-07nov.pdf

NCT (2017) 'Reviews of evidence', https://www.nct.org.uk/professional/research/reviews-evidence

Parliament UK (2011) 'Evidence-based policy', https://www.publications.parliament.uk/pa/ld201012/ldselect/ldsctech/179/17907.htm

Research Excellence Framework (2014) 'About the REF', www.ref.ac.uk/about

Conclusion

Sally Dowling, David Pontin and Kate Boyer

Introduction

This edited volume brings together work from the 'core participant' attendees at the UK ESRC-funded seminar series 'Social experiences of breastfeeding: building bridges between research and policy', which ran during 2015 and 2016. We wanted to share some of the dialogue and enthusiasm with people who could use it in their everyday life/work supporting women who breastfeed their babies. Each academic contributor (authors of the section chapters) presented their work during one of the six seminars. Most of the UK-based presenters also attended and took part in the other seminars, so we had an ongoing conversation over the life of the series.

Some of the policy/practice contributors (authors of the section commentary pieces) also presented work at a seminar. The others attended most of the events, and they have provided insight and reflection into the usefulness of the academic work for policy makers and practitioners. We have interpreted 'practitioner' in the widest sense, and use it to refer to breastfeeding support delivered by health professionals, breastfeeding peer and other supporters, infant feeding leads in NHS hospitals/community services, and local authority managers.

The chapters in this book build on the seminar presentations themselves (edited audio recordings are available via the seminar series website if you want to get a flavour of the atmosphere). When we were planning the book, we grouped the chapters together and linked them with the commentators. There were many different versions before we settled on this arrangement, as there are many connections between chapters in different sections, and across the book. In this conclusion, we make some of these links; there are many others that readers will draw themselves, and we'd be happy to hear from you to continue the conversation.

The seminar series, and this book, set out to address the following questions:

- How does attending to the micro-practices and affective and embodied experiences of breastfeeding women advance extant knowledge about the reasons for breastfeeding cessation?
- How can we further understanding about inequalities in breastfeeding rates by focusing on the nuances of day-to-day breastfeeding?
- How might an increased understanding of these perspectives influence policy?

Connections between disciplines and across continents

When we were planning the bid to the ESRC for funding, we wanted to bring together social science researchers and scholars from other traditions and disciplines to think about the social experiences of breastfeeding. There is work here from sociologists, psychologists, anthropologists and geographers, alongside academics from English and cultural studies, nursing and public health, media and communication, environmental studies and law. We think this marks the book out as different when compared with recent breastfeeding publications, although it builds on Smith, Hausman and Labbok's (2012) book that came out of the 5th Breastfeeding and Feminism Symposium (now called the Breastfeeding and Feminism International Conference, BFIC).

These annual symposia/conferences have been run by Paige Hall Smith and the late, influential Miriam Labbok at the University of North Carolina, Chapel Hill, United States. Several of the chapter authors in this collection and other seminar speakers also authored chapters in that 2012 book following their presentations at the 5th symposium (Sally Dowling, David Pontin, Fiona Giles, Dawn Leeming and Abigail Locke), and many contributors to this volume refer to its chapters. Other contributors to this book have been involved in the Breastfeeding and Feminism events as speakers (Cecilia Tomori, Danielle Groleau and Maia Boswell-Penc), and we celebrated this link by inviting Paige Hall Smith to attend the final seminar to share her experiences of running a successful series linking academics with policy makers and practitioners. Paige's talk is on the seminar series website and we are hoping to continue our connection with BFIC in the future.

You'll have noticed that the academic contributors in this volume are mostly from the UK, and the majority of them work in UK universities. We also have contributions from Australia (Alison Bartlett and Fiona Giles) and the US (Maia Boswell-Penc and Cecilia Tomori, who is now at Durham University in the UK). This combination provided us with some interesting comparative perspectives, as well as raising issues that are truly cross–global (for example, Fiona Giles' discussion of 'brelfies'). The seminar series therefore ran in the UK with an international backdrop. We know from the literature that many of the issues we explored through the seminars are also relevant to people living and working in other developed countries, and we hope this volume speaks to them too.

We were very pleased to support several PhD students and early career researchers through the work of the seminar series. Some of them were able to come regularly to the seminars as attendees, and some also presented their work: Melanie Fraser early in the seminar series, and LulaMecinska, Sharon Tugwell, Gretel Finch and Laura Streeter at the final event. For various reasons we couldn't include all their work here, but we appreciate their commitment, involvement and contributions to the seminar series and wish them well for the future.

Policy and practice contributions

We wanted to think about how academic work on breastfeeding could be used in practice, and whether it could influence policy in some way. The commentary piece authors (Nicki Symes, Geraldine Lucas, Sally Tedstone, Sally Johnson, Emma Laird and Elizabeth Mayo) work in a variety of settings with breastfeeding women and practitioners (in the widest sense) who support them. Some commission services for breastfeeding women, some train midwives and contribute to the professional debates around this, and some work as breastfeeding peer supporters. We value their input to the seminar series, and their perspective on the academic work presented here is a valuable counterweight in helping us to achieve our aims. We have only been able to elicit the views of a small number of people who attended the series in this way. However, throughout our seminar series we wanted to acknowledge and value the insight gained from involving policy and practice colleagues who presented their work in the 'policy/practice' slot at each seminar, as well as those who attended the seminar series as participants and contributed to the discussions and the networking components.

Funding a place for an NCT (a large UK parenting charity) attendee at every seminar session also contributed to the series aim, and their participation was invaluable (continuing here with Elizabeth Mayo's input). We were fortunate to have a number of attendees from senior positions in the breastfeeding field operating at national and international levels. They generously shared with us their insights into the issues and provided a context to some of the other discussions. Francesca Entwistle and Fiona Dykes (authors of the UK policy/ practice context piece), and Sally Tedstone (author of the series context piece) were all members of our 'core participants' group, and were invaluable in reviewing and evaluating what we did from their perspectives as practitioners/policy makers/participants.

The academic contribution of this book

Francesca Entwistle and Fiona Dykes' policy context piece provides a background against which the academic can be interpreted. Complementary chapters by Dawn Leeming and Lisa Smyth follow on by addressing affective and embodied experiences through their discussions of emotional intensity in breastfeeding promotion and managing shame in breastfeeding support. Their disciplinary approaches of sociology and psychology, respectively, provide different but complementary perspectives.

Leeming explores and analyses shame and breastfeeding experiences, focusing on a discussion of shame versus guilt. Of particular use for practitioners, the chapter discusses shame resilience, paying attention to the dynamics of shame and how these can be used when planning and providing emotional support to mothers. There is scope for future work here in developing work practices and training for practitioners, and working on local policies to build shame resilience strategies. Smyth also reminds us of the connections between inequalities and breastfeeding, and links them to status anxiety, pride and shame. She highlights the interrelationship between shame and pride experienced by many mothers, and relates it to breastfeeding advocacy and the urgent need for it to be addressed by health policy.

The diverse range of affective and embodied experiences are addressed by Fiona Giles' work on 'brelfies', Alison Bartlett's piece about Skywhale, and the chapters written by Sally Dowling and Cecilia Tomori on long-term breastfeeding and night-time feeding, respectively. Giles and Bartlett take a very different focus to Smyth and Leeming. They stimulate us to consider quite different thinking about women's experiences of breastfeeding, about it's connection with the social and the maternal, considering controversial images of things or events and the response evoked from/in us towards the thing portrayed. Some of this territory and thinking may be unfamiliar and challenging to readers from a policy and practice background. In her endpiece reflection on the seminars, Sally Tedstone points out that some of the seminar presentations did not always use accessible language considering the diversity present in a 'mixed' audience of practitioners, policy makers and academics. We acknowledge Sally's view, but in defence, we think these chapters are important for a book like this because they present ideas in engaging and stimulating ways, and they make them available to a wider readership. The challenge here is for all of us to translate across traditions and work practice boundaries.

Running through the book are examples of the 'nuances' and micro-practices attended to by women in their day-to-day experiences of breastfeeding. These are diverse and range from migrant mothers' experiences and the notion of lost milk (Louise Condon), the liminality of women who breastfeed long term (Sally Dowling), mothers returning to work and wanting to continue breastfeeding (Melanie Fraser), the impact of sleeping practices and night-time breastfeeding (Cecilia Tomori), and the shifting divide of breastfeeding in private and in public (Fiona Giles). Together these chapters provide a deeper understanding of what breastfeeding is *like* for women, how they make decisions about what to do and when, how they communicate their decisions to other people, and how they present themselves to the world in relation to the decisions they have made. Giles also relates this to policy and practice by thinking about the consciousness-raising function of 'brelfies', and the 'critical area of advocacy' of breastfeeding in public. Both Tomori and Giles provide useful historical/contemporary contexts: Tomori in the form of a historical review of US night-time breastfeeding, and Giles by reviewing the history of the 'brelfie'.

We wanted to think more about inequalities in breastfeeding rates by considering these 'nuances of day-to-day breastfeeding'. Condon's chapter specifically focuses on women who are migrants to the UK who find themselves living in precarious social and financial conditions. Her chapter highlights the challenges for breastfeeding promotion in understanding the subtleties of lives that may be different to those of practitioners and policy makers. The need to understand the context in which infant feeding decisions are made is also highlighted in Tomori's exploration of night-time feeding practice and Smyth's focus on data from Northern Ireland, where breastfeeding rates are very low compared to other developed countries.

Critical responses to how women are advised and supported around breastfeeding run through a number of chapters. Locke develops a critique of breastfeeding promotion and the influence of neoliberal political philosophy, while Brown draws attention to the subtext present in parenting literature and its allure for new parents in their attempt to make the transition to parenthood. Newell focuses on how a practice-based approach can be useful in understanding the gap between policy and practice, and ways in which policy may be developed to support practice, while Fraser looks at breastfeeding and work from the perspective of employers using insights from legal analysis.

Ways in which we can develop a deeper understanding about the cessation of breastfeeding, particularly in the context of the Unicef Call to Action, and the ways in which the recent focus has been on the importance of normalising breastfeeding (Unicef, 2016; Lancet, 2016), are addressed by a thread that runs through many of the chapters. Leeming, Smyth, Dowling and Condon write about normalising women's feelings, breastfeeding at different ages and different cultural experiences of breastfeeding. The impact of policy and of legal frameworks (Newell and Fraser) and the influence of the media and publications (Brown and Locke) are also addressed and constitute part of this strand. What actually happens in families and how this impacts on continuing to breastfeed is discussed (see Tomori, Dowling and Condon), as well as the images that contribute to how breastfeeding and breasts are seen (Bartlett and Giles), and the pervasive messages to which all mothers are subject in their everyday lives (Locke and Brown).

Our seminar series was established on the premise that breastfeeding and supporting women to breastfeed are worthwhile and valuable activities for individual women, their babies and their families, and for society at large. However, in constructing the series in the way that we did, we also created a space for critical thinking, and for questioning and challenging people's perceptions of breastfeeding promotion and support. Abigail Locke provides a critical social psychology perspective on breastfeeding promotion, while Amy Brown critiques the support that women can gain from parenting books and how this might influence the practice of breastfeeding and continuing to breastfeed. The broader cultural expectations about what is considered to be normal in terms of food production and infant feeding are also discussed in Maia Boswell-Penc's work.

Finally, we are pleased that our cross-disciplinary perspectives also bring with them different ways of using social science theory to think about breastfeeding experiences – explorations of status inequality, shame resilience, liminality, affect and the idea of the matrixial are some of these. As editors and coordinators of the seminar series, we find it interesting that our commentary writers have been both challenged and enthused by some of these ideas, and hope that a wider audience will find them useful when looking at their own practice and the situations in which they work.

Our influence on policy and practice

Breastfeeding in developed countries can be seen to be a wicked problem (Rittel and Webber, 1973) or a social mess (Horn, 2001). A social mess is constrained by closely woven social, political, technological and economic aspects – making it hard to grasp the phenomenon. It is not a simple problem with an immediate solution. It is complicated and ambiguous, constructed differently depending on one's world view, and value-based conflicts are likely. This leads to uncertainty about initial conditions and location, and about appropriate actions that may be taken.

In editing this book, we did not set out to advocate a simple solution for a complex problem; rather, we see the seminar series and the production of the book as small steps to building solutions to complex situations. One of our original questions was, 'How might an increased understanding of these [academic, social science] perspectives influence policy?' In short, our answer is, 'We don't know because it is a wicked problem.' We are clear that we have had some impact on practice, as our commentators have noted this (see the commentaries for Parts I and II, specifically) along with the feedback that we had from those practitioners who attended seminars. In publishing this book, we share the authors' insights with a wider unknown public, and we hope that the authors will continue to influence the field through their continued study of these issues, and also through the connections they made at the seminars.

The links between Chapters One and Two, and policy and practice, are picked up on by Sally Johnson and Sally Tedstone (in the commentary for Part I), who chose to write the majority of their piece about the issue of shame, their increased understanding of this, and its meaning for their work. In doing so, they focus on some of the practical ways in which they could introduce these ideas into their sphere of influence – through the development of a group for women who are experiencing significant breastfeeding challenges, and by encouraging and focusing on more personalised and woman-centred care, provided by people with better attuned 'shame antennae'. This notion of shame antennae has profound implications for the initial training and continued professional development for all people working with mothers of young babies. In the commentary for Part III, Nicki Symes, Elizabeth Mayo and Emma Laird also pick up on this, and link Giles' point about changing the perception of breasts from sexual to maternal with Bartlett's argument about the importance of the normalisation of breastfeeding for the benefit of babies, women and society in general. Together these ideas have the potential to shape and mould policy direction to meet women's needs and the needs of society.

Conclusion

Back in 2013 when we first entertained the idea for this project, we hoped that the work of applying for and securing the ESRC seminar series funding was just the beginning of something bigger. Looking back on events and reflecting on running the seminar series and producing this edited collection, we think that it was. The seminar series has acted as an incubator and several collaborations are emerging. We have 'joined the conversation' (Unicef, 2016), individually and collectively, through this book and through seminar members' representation at meetings of the All-Party Parliamentary Group on Infant Feeding and Inequalities (see the Introduction). Our aim of building bridges has begun, and we are confident that the relationships we built over the course of the seminar series will continue to span the world and contribute to resolving the wicked problem of how can we help women to breastfeed their babies.

References

Horn, R. (2001) 'Knowledge mapping for complex social messes': a presentation to Foundations in the Knowledge Economy at the David and Lucile Packard Foundation, 16 July 2001, https://nautilus.org/gps/solving/social-messes-robert-e-horn

Lancet (2016) 'Editorial: breastfeeding: achieving the new normal', *Lancet*, 376: 404.

Rittel, H.W.J. and Webber, M. M. (1973) 'Dilemmas in a general theory of planning', *Policy Sciences*, 4(2): 155–69.

Smith, P. H., Hausman, B. and Labbok, M. (eds) (2012) *Beyond health, beyond choice: Breastfeeding constraints and realities*, New Brunswick, NJ: Rutgers University Press.

Unicef (2016) 'Protecting health and saving lives: A call to action', https://www.unicef.org.uk/babyfriendly/wp-content/uploads/sites/2/2016/04/Call-to-Action-Unicef-UK-Baby-Friendly-Initiative.pdf

Appendix:
Schedule for ESRC Seminar Series:
Social Experiences of Breastfeeding:
Building bridges between research
and policy, 2015–16

Date	Venue	Theme	Presenter 1	Presenter 2	Presenter 3	Presenter 4
11 March 2015	The Watershed Bristol	Breastfeeding and changing cultures of parenting	Dr Cecilia Tomori, Johns Hopkins Bloomberg School of Public Health, US	Dr Amy Brown, Swansea University, UK	Dr Lisa Smyth, Queens University Belfast, UK	Sally Tedstone, National Breastfeeding Programme Co-ordinator, Public Health Wales, UK
1 June 2015	Cardiff University	Breastfeeding, affect and materiality	Prof. Alison Bartlett, University Western Australia, Australia	Dr Kate Boyer, Cardiff University, UK	Dr Lucila Newell, Sussex University, UK	Nicki Symes, Breastfeeding Co-ordinator, Bristol City Council, UK
4 Nov 2015	UWE Bristol	Breastfeeding, wage work and social exclusion	Dr Danielle Groleau, McGill University, Canada	Dr Melanie Fraser (then PhD Student), UWE, UK	Prof. Louise Condon, Swansea University, UK	April Whincop, Barnardo's Breastfeeding Peer Support Co-ordinator, Bristol, UK
2 March 2016	Cardiff University	Breastfeeding and the politics of embodiment	Dr Maia Boswell-Penc, Independent researcher, NY, US	Dr Dawn Leeming, Huddersfield University, UK	Dr Sally Dowling, UWE, UK	Geraldine Lucas, UWE, UK
9 June 2016	National Museum Cardiff	Breastfeeding, media and popular culture	Dr Fiona Giles, University of Sydney, Australia	Dr Catherine Angell, Bournemouth University, UK	Prof. Abigail Locke, Bradford University, UK	Prof Shantini Paranjothy, Cardiff University, UK
9 Nov 2016	The Watershed Bristol	Thinking innovatively about breastfeeding policy	Prof. Fiona Dykes, University of Central Lancashire, UK	Francesca Entwistle, Hertfordshire University/ Professional Advisor, UNICEF UK Baby Friendly Initiative, UK	Short presentations	Hollie McNish Performance Poet, UK

Short presentations: Prof. Paige Hall Smith, University of North Carolina, Greensboro, US; PhD students: Laura Streeter (London School of Hygiene and Tropical Medicine), Lula Mecinksa (Lancaster University), and Sharon Tugwell (Birkbeck College, London); Early career researcher: Gretel Finch (Bristol University)

Note: Some contributors have changed jobs and/or institutions since the presentations listed here were given. Please see the list of contributors at the beginning of the book for information correct at the time of going to press.

Index